Physiotherapy Management of Haemophilia

Physiotherapy Management of Haemophilia

EDITED BY

Brenda Buzzard

Superintendent Physiotherapist
The Newcastle Upon Tyne Hospitals NHS Trust
Northern Regional Haemophilia Service
Royal Victoria Infirmary, Newcastle upon Tyne

AND

Karen Beeton

Senior Lecturer
Department of Physiotherapy
University of Hertfordshire, Hatfield
Honorary Lecturer
Royal Free and University College Medical School
University College, London

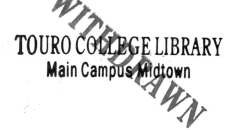

Blackwell
Science

MT

First published 2000

Set by BookEns Ltd, Royston, Herts
Printed and bound in Great Britain
by MPG Books Ltd, Bodmin, Cornwall

The Blackwell Science logo is a
trade mark of Blackwell Science Ltd,
registered at the United Kingdom
Trade Marks Registry

For further information on
Blackwell Science, visit our website:
www.blackwell-science.com

DISTRIBUTORS

Marston Book Services Ltd
PO Box 269
Abingdon, Oxon OX14 4YN
(*Orders*: Tel: 01235 465500
Fax: 01235 465555)
USA
Blackwell Science, Inc.
Commerce Place
350 Main Street
Malden, MA 02148-5018
(*Orders*: Tel: 800 759 6102
781 388 8250
Fax: 781 388 8255)
Canada
Login Brothers Book Company
324 Saulteaux Crescent
Winnipeg, Manitoba R3J 3T2
(*Orders*: Tel: 204 837 2987)

Australia
Blackwell Science Pty Ltd
54 University Street
Carlton, Victoria 3053
(*Orders*: Tel: 3 9347 0300
Fax: 3 9347 5001)

A catalogue record for this title
is available from the British Library

ISBN 0-632-05764-5

Library of Congress
Cataloging-in-publication Data
Physiotherapy management of haemophilia
/edited by Brenda Buzzard and
Karen Beeton.
    p.   cm.
Includes bibliographical references and
    index.
ISBN 0-632-05764-5
1. Musculoskeletal system–
Diseases–Physical therapy.
2. Hemophilia–Complications–Physical
therapy. I. Buzzard, Brenda. II. Beeton,
Karen. [DNLM: 1 Hemophilia A-
rehabilitation.
2. Arthralgia–therapy. 3. Contracture-
therapy.
4. Hemarthrosis–therapy. 5. Physical
Therapy–methods. 6. Synovitis-
therapy. WH 325 P578 2000]
RC925.5.P47 2000
616.1′57206515–dc21   00-039740

2/24/06

Contents

List of Contributors

Caroline Barmatz BSc PT
Hydrotherapy Department, Supervisor, The Chaim Sheba Medical Center, Tel Hashomer Hospital, Israel

Karen Beeton MPhty BSc(Hons) MCSP
Senior Lecturer, Department of Physiotherapy, University of Hertfordshire, Hatfield, UK; and Honorary Lecturer, Royal Free and University College Medical School, University College, London, UK

Brenda M. Buzzard MSc PostGradDip MCSP
Superintendent Physiotherapist, The Newcastle Upon Tyne Hospitals NHS Trust, Northern Regional Haemophilia Service, Royal Victoria Infirmary, Newcastle upon Tyne, UK

Andrew Clements MCSP
Physiotherapist to Leicester Haemophilia Comprehensive Care Centre, Leicester Royal Infirmary NHS Trust, Leicester; and Associate Clinical Teacher Leicester University, Faculty of Medicine, Leicester, UK

Jane Cornwell MCSP
Physiotherapiest c/o Chartered Society of Physiotherapy, 14 Bedford Row, London WC1R 4ED

Mandy Higginbottom MCSP
Superintendent Physiotherapist, Physiotherapy Department, Royal Hallamshire Hospital, Glossop Road, Sheffield, UK

Lily Heijnen MD PhD
Van Creveld Kliniek UMC Utrecht, Rehabilitation Centre De Trappenberg Huizen, The Netherlands

Piet de Kleijn PT
Physiotherapist, Department of Rehabilitation and Nutritional Sciences, Faculty of Medicine, Van Creveld Clinic, University Medical Center, Utrecht, The Netherlands

Nico L.U. van Meeteren PhD

Associate Professor, Division Rehabilitation and Nutritional Sciences; Staff member of the Rudolf Magnus Institute for Neurosciences, University Medical Center, Utrecht, The Netherlands

Victoria Leckie MCSP

Senior Physiotherapist, Royal Hallamshire Hospital, Sheffield, UK

Lucy Orr MCSP

Physiotherapy Specialist in Haemophilia, The Haemophilia Reference Centre, St Thomas' Hospital, Lambeth Palace Road, London SE1 7EH, UK

Jane Padkin MCSP

Superintendent Physiotherapist III, Physiotherapy Department, Royal Free Hospital, Pond Street, London NW3 2QG, UK

E. Carlos Rodriguez-Merchan MD PhD

Consultant Orthopaedic Surgeon, Haemophilia Centre, La Paz University Hospital, Madrid, Spain

Dionne Ryder MSc MCSP

Senior Lecturer, Department of Physiotherapy, University of Hertfordshire, Hatfield, UK

Mohammed Tariq Sohail MBBS (Pb), MCh.orth (L'Pool), FRCS (Ed), FRCS (GIGS), FICS

Post Graduate Medical Institute, Lahore General Hospital, Lahore, Pakistan

David Stephensen

Physiotherapist, Kent Haemophilia Centre, Kent and Canterbury Hospital, Ethelbert Road, Canterbury CT1 3NG, UK

Rochelle Tiktinsky BSc PT

The National Hemophilia Center, The Chaim Sheba Medical Center, Tel Hashomer Hospital, Israel

Forewords

Haemophilia is a lifelong inherited bleeding disorder character-ized by severe, spontaneous bleeding resulting in chronic, pain-ful joint deformities. Without treatment, individuals with haemophilia will die in childhood or early life. The development of safe and effective clotting factor concentrates has enabled newly diagnosed children with haemophilia to be treated safely with prophylaxis, or regular injections with clotting factor con-centrate, to stop bleeds, particularly joint bleeds.

However, there is a generation of patients with haemophilia who had poor treatment in their childhood and now have major joint disability requiring physiotherapy support and often sur-gical intervention with joint replacements. In the developed world, high purity concentrates have enabled peri-operative delivery of concentrate factor by continuous infusion, which gives added safety, not only for the period of surgery, but also for the period of more intensive physiotherapy postoperatively.

In contrast, it has been suggested that 80% of those with haemophilia in the world do not have access to adequate medical care. Many of such individuals are undiagnosed, untreated and therefore suffer enormously. Although expertise of orthopaedic care cannot always be provided for such patients because of the constraint of lack of clotting factor provision for economic reasons, physiotherapy is a relatively less expensive option. Fortunately in the less resourced parts of the world, the provision of skilled personnel is sometimes better than in the so-called developed world because of the relatively lower salary paid. Consequently, as a generation of children grows up on prophylaxis, healthcare professionals will have much to learn from their more experi-enced counterparts in the less resourced countries.

The patient with haemophilia presents a particular challenge for those providing musculoskeletal care: quality of life can be transformed by such care. We all hope that there is a generation of children with haemophilia growing up who will not have musculoskeletal problems — but until then, this comprehensive book *Physiotherapy Management of Haemophilia* will provide a useful reference for those providing physiotherapy care with the comprehensive care team.

Professor Christine Lee
Haemophilia Centre and Haemostasis Unit,
Royal Free Hospital, UK

Despite the extraordinary advances in the haematological prophylaxis and treatment of haemophilia, the musculoskeletal problems of this condition are still very common. Only 20–30% of the world population have access to adequate haematological management, mainly because of the high cost of replacement products. It has been demonstrated that with prophylaxis from 2 to 18 years, severe haemophilia can be transformed into mild haemophilia. Thus, in the developed countries, orthopaedic surgery is less often required in persons with haemophilia, although it is still necessary from time to time. Although I am the only orthopaedic surgeon operating on these patients in Spain, the musculoskeletal treatment of haemophilia only takes 5% of my professional time. On the contrary, in those countries without adequate economic resources, the orthopaedic complications of haemophilia still continue the same as they did 25 years ago.

The main complications of haemophilia from the musculoskeletal perspective include: haemarthroses, synovitis, articular flexion contractures, axial malalignment of the limbs, haematomas, pseudotumours and haemophilic arthropathy. All of these can lead to painful episodes and also to a progressive multiarticular disability, with tremendous psychological, family and professional implications. In my opinion, the ideal treatment of musculoskeletal problems in haemophilia should include:

1 an early and continuous haematological prophylaxis to try to avoid haemorrhages;

2 an aggressive haematological treatment of bleeding episodes when they occur;

3 the immediate aspiration of articular bleedings as soon as they are detected;

4 the early performance of procedures for synovial destruction (synoviorthesis, arthroscopic synovectomy, open surgical synovectomy) as soon as a synovitis is diagnosed;
5 an early and aggressive rehabilitation programme to avoid the development of fixed articular contractures.

Physiotherapy is particularly important in the prevention of fixed articular contractures which if left untreated will require further orthopaedic procedures. The importance of postoperative physiotherapy, after synovectomies, tendon lengthening or tendon releases, osteotomies, joint arthroplasties and surgical removal of pseudotumours must also be emphasized.

The close co-operation between physiotherapists, physicians specialized in rehabilitation and orthopaedic surgeons is paramount for the adequate treatment of musculoskeletal problems in haemophilia today. In my opinion, there has been, and there still is, a fruitful intellectual co-operation between myself, and Brenda Buzzard and Karen Beeton within the endeavour of the World Federation of Haemophilia. There is no doubt that such a long-lasting co-operation is the reason why the co-editors of this book have invited me to write this Foreword. I am sure that this excellent book, with well-known contributors from the UK and the rest of the world, will be of great value in the understanding of the most recent concepts in the physiotherapy management of haemophilia. The benefit will be not only for physiotherapists, but also for physicians specializing in rehabilitation, rheumatologists, orthopaedic surgeons and haematologists interested in the treatment of such a devastating condition. I am sure that its contents will give fruitful physiotherapy information for many years. The editors and contributors to this book are to be congratulated. We will gain immeasurably from this compilation of timely advances, enabling us to better serve our haemophilia patients.

E. Carlos Rodriguez-Merchan MD PhD
Haemophilia Centre, La Paz University Hospital, Spain

Preface

The management of haemophilia has changed enormously over the last 30 years. Prior to the widespread availability of factor replacement, patients suffered many bleeds in the musculo-skeletal system and subsequently developed arthropathy affecting multiple joints. Today the outlook is more optimistic. Early and adequate treatment of bleeds and prophylactic programmes has ensured that recovery of bleeds is more complete and the devastating effects of arthropathy are minimized. Despite these developments many patients still present with bleeds, chronic synovitis and arthropathy due to inadequately treated bleeds in the past and therefore physiotherapy remains an important aspect of treatment.

Alongside these changes has been the development of the physiotherapy profession. Physiotherapists have increasing responsibility for the management of their patients and also have an increasing array of concepts and modalities with which to treat patients with haemophilia.

This book aims to provide a comprehensive overview of physiotherapy treatment concepts and management strategies currently available that can be incorporated into the management programmes for patients with haemophilia. It has been written by physiotherapists with a broad range of experience of haemophilia based on their clinical experience and supported by evidence from the literature when available.

We hope that this book will be useful in providing new ideas for physiotherapists who regularly treat patients with haemophilia as well as a source of reference for those who may only treat a few patients. We also hope that it will be a valuable source of information for other members of the comprehensive care team, the doctors, nurses, orthopaedic surgeons and counsellors who are also involved in managing these patients. Overall our ultimate aim is that this book will highlight the vital role that physiotherapy can play in the care of these patients in improving musculoskeletal function.

Brenda Buzzard
Karen Beeton

Acknowledgements

The editors would like to acknowledge the generous support of the following pharmaceutical companies and organizations which has made the publication of this book possible.

World Federation of Haemophilia
Griffols UK Ltd
Bio Products Laboratory
Aventis Behring
Haemophilia Chartered Physiotherapists Association
Baxter Healthcare Ltd
Bayer PLC
Aircast UK
Physio Med Services Ltd

1 Principles of Assessment in Haemophilia

Karen Beeton and Dionne Ryder

The manifestations of severe haemophilia include spontaneous bleeding into joints and muscles, with joints accounting for 80% of all bleeding episodes [1]. Left untreated, the effects of chronic synovitis and disabling chronic arthropathy are all too apparent with severe pain, deformity, loss of range of movement and decreased function. Physiotherapists, as part of the comprehensive care team, can assist the haemophilic patient in restoring or improving musculoskeletal function. Haemophilia is a relatively rare disease with Haemophilia A having a prevalence of one in 10 000 males and Haemophilia B with a prevalence of one in 50 000 [2]. Patients may live a considerable distance from their major comprehensive care centre where a named physiotherapist may be responsible for their physiotherapy care. They may therefore, need to seek physiotherapy treatment at a local hospital. Thus it is essential that all physiotherapists have an understanding of the underlying condition so that these patients can be managed in an optimal way. Prior to identifying management strategies or undertaking treatment, a thorough assessment is essential. This chapter will describe the principles of the subjective and physical examination with relevance to the patient with haemophilia.

Subjective examination

The main focus of the subjective examination is for the patient to outline the problem for which they are seeking treatment from their own perspective. For the physiotherapist, the skill in identifying relevant information requires 'care, patience and a critical attitude' [3]. Clinical reasoning is an integral part of this process and has been defined as 'the thinking skills and knowledge used to make clinical decisions and judgements through the evaluation, diagnosis and management of a patient problem' [4].

The main aims of the subjective examination are to:
- establish baseline information regarding the patient's haemophilia status;
- determine the source of the symptoms and/or dysfunction;
- identify any factors which may be contributing to the specific problem;
- determine whether there are any precautions or contraindications to the physical examination or treatment; and
- to establish the history of the specific problem [4].

Baseline information regarding the patient's haemophilia status

It is important at the outset to establish the type of bleeding disorder, the level of circulating factor, whether the patient is on prophylaxis or 'on demand' treatment, route of infusion and the presence of inhibitors. Patients with circulating factor levels < 1iu/dL are severely affected and therefore need to be handled prudently in order to avoid causing a bleed. Patients with inhibitors need particular care in management, as medical options are more limited and uncontrolled bleeding can be life threatening [2,5].

If factor replacement is required prior to physiotherapy intervention, it is important to confirm that it has been administered. If the patient is on prophylaxis, the timing of the prophylaxis needs to be established. The half life of Factor VIII is 8 hours and for Factor IX is 18 hours [2] indicating that after this time there is only half of the circulating factor that was administered, therefore the risks of bleeding are greater.

The source of symptoms and/or dysfunction

Patients with haemophilia may present with musculoskeletal problems directly relating to their haemophilia or they may complain of other musculoskeletal problems, such as back pain, neck pain or sporting injuries commonly seen in the general population.

The patient's age, occupation and hobbies should be identified as they often impact on the setting of appropriate goals and, ultimately, the prognosis. A body chart can be useful in providing a clear record of the area and type of symptoms the patient is experiencing [6]. The distribution, type, depth and severity of pain, and the relationship of pain to any other symptoms which may be present such as weakness, giving way, locking, numbness and paraesthesia, can help to identify possible structures at fault [7]. Pain of a mechanical origin tends to be intermittent and related to movements in one or more directions. Pain due to inflammatory causes may be constant although fluctuating in intensity, with prolonged morning stiffness and exacerbated by rest [8]. Analysis of the symptoms provides initial hypotheses regarding the source of symptoms or dysfunction as well as having implications for possible management strategies and also prognosis.

An initial hypothesis of the source of symptoms in a haemophilic patient who presents with acute onset of groin pain associated with numbness over the anterior thigh may be an iliopsoas haematoma. Other diagnoses which would have to be considered are a hip bleed, retroperitoneal bleed or even appendicitis [9].

Arthropathy may be the initial hypothesis for a patient who presents with persistent pain over the shoulder joint described as a nagging ache. However, it is important to remember that the area of symptoms does not necessarily identify the structures at fault [6]. Pain can be referred from a more proximal site and the relevant spinal region should always be checked to exclude its involvement [6]. Having developed an initial hypothesis or hypotheses, the remaining subjective questions will add further support to the hypothesis or result in the physiotherapist considering other options.

Once the symptoms have been described it is essential to identify how the symptoms behave and establish the aggravating and easing factors for each of the symptoms. This will determine the severity and the irritability of the condition. Identifying the severity and irritability accurately will ensure that the vigour of the physical examination is appropriate for the disorder as well as being useful reassessment markers in evaluating the effectiveness of the treatment [7].

The severity of symptoms relates to both the intensity of

symptoms experienced and how much the symptoms interfere with daily activities. Intensity may be assessed using a visual analogue scale. Irritability is defined as how easily symptoms are provoked and how long they take to settle [3]. If the condition is deemed to be severe and/or irritable, the scope of the physical examination will need to be restricted and particular attention given to careful and precise manual handling procedures in order to avoid exacerbating symptoms.

The behaviour of symptoms over 24 hours, e.g. night, morning and end of day will often give additional clues as to the underlying disorder. Arthropathy of a joint often presents with initial pain and stiffness in the morning which improves with light activity and increases again with prolonged or weight-bearing activities. Functional activities relating to the patient's work, ability to climb stairs, driving, walking distance and use of aids such as sticks or crutches and appliances such as chair lifts or additional rails also needs to be established. Some patients may need more probing questions to identify the key problems. The restriction to the lifestyle of the adult with haemophilia can often be very marked. This may be due to the presence of advanced haemophilic arthropathy affecting multiple joints, as a result of inadequately treated bleeds in the past when factor concentrates were not so readily available.

Contributing factors

Factors which may contribute to the ongoing maintenance of symptoms may include physical factors such as poor working postures (e.g. when using a computer), poor technique at sport (e.g. inappropriate racquet grip or inadequate footwear), or other factors such as leg length inequality [4]. Psychosocial factors such as depression or anxiety and attitudes to haemophilia may also impact on the response to treatment [4,10]. Insufficient attention to these issues will reduce the benefits of treatment and may lead to poor outcomes or recurrence of symptoms.

Precautions and contraindications

Part of the role of the subjective is to identify any precautions or contraindications to physiotherapy management and thus referral of the patient for further investigations. Enquiries should be made regarding the patient's general health, weight, drug therapy, results of X-rays and other medical investigations [6].

In patients who are stereopositive for the human immunodeficiency virus (HIV), apparently benign musculo-skeletal presentations may be due to septic arthritis or the effects of drug management. Septic arthritis has been reported more commonly since the occurrence of HIV in the haemophilic population. The knee, elbow and ankles were identified as the most commonly affected joints [11,12]. Diagnosis was made due to marked pain, lack of response to factor replacement and pyrexia.

A lack of improvement following factor replacement may also indicate the development of inhibitors to Factor VIII or IX [5,13]. If the physiotherapist has any concerns that the patient may have a nonmusculoskeletal cause of symptoms, this should be discussed with the appropriate medical personnel prior to any intervention.

Information should also be sought regarding analgesic usage either in the short or longer term. A reduction in medication can also be a marker indicating improvement in the underlying condition. An acute bleed or arthropathy can be extremely painful and adequate analgesia must be prescribed [13] although, interestingly, chronic synovitis of a joint following recurrent bleeds is not usually associated with pain.

The history of the specific problem

Information regarding the history of the specific problem, its onset either spontaneous or traumatic, whether factor replacement was given and the response to treatment should be identified. It is also necessary to establish whether the condition is improving, staying the same or worsening. It is particularly important to be vigilant when managing the patient with haemophilia where an acute bleed has followed a traumatic incident. In this case the bleed may appear to be the focus of the problem but may in fact mask a fracture.

Past medical history should include discussion of recent joint or muscle bleeds, joints which have been subjected to recurrent bleeds, the so called 'target joint', previous physiotherapy and response, and any previous surgical interventions.

Summary

At the conclusion of the subjective examination the physio-therapist will have identified the severity, irritability and possible hypotheses regarding the structures or dysfunction involved. Due to the difficulties in identifying specific structures, con-clusive structural differentiation may not be possible [4] and the physiotherapist may have to develop a working hypothesis rather than a specific diagnosis [6].

Physical examination

The aim of the physical examination is to specifically test struc-tures in a systematic order to confirm or refute the hypotheses generated during the subjective examination. It is essential that the physiotherapist uses information from the subjective and physical examination in an open minded manner and this requires continuous clinical reasoning and analysis of exam-ination findings [14]. When performing assessment procedures on a patient with haemophilia, particular care must be employed at all times in order to avoid causing a bleed or exacerbating symptoms.

During the physical examination the physiotherapist will be eliciting information concerning:

1 what the patient feels during specific tests, which requires clear communication with the patient throughout the examina-tion;

2 responses that can be measured by the physiotherapist, i.e. joint range of movement or muscle strength.

The components of the examination [6]

The main components of the physical examination include:
- observation;
- joint tests;
- muscle tests;
- neurological examination;
- other tests;
- palpation.

Observation

Informal assessment of the functional status of a patient begins from the moment the physiotherapist meets the patient. This can be formally assessed further by asking the patient to demonstrate a specific functional activity, i.e. walking, climbing the stairs or sitting to standing. This will allow the physiotherapist to ascertain the nature and extent of their disability. More specifically, the physiotherapist should examine the patient's static posture in order to observe any postural abnormalities and categorize the postural type [15]. An increased lordosis may be apparent which might be associated with a flexion contracture of the knee or occur following an iliopsoas bleed [9,16].

Joint tests

The joint tests include the testing of active and passive physiological movements and passive accessory movements. The aim of the joint tests is to reproduce the patient's symptoms, i.e. find a comparable sign [3], determine the quality, pattern, range and pain response for each movement, and obtain markers which can be used for reassessment purposes.

Active physiological movements. Prior to any movement the patient's symptoms should be established. Active physiological movements are assessed before passive movements. The movements most likely to be painful should be performed last to prevent symptoms persisting during subsequent movements. If the patient's contralateral side is unaffected, this can indicate the normal for that patient. The physiotherapist will note the willingness of the patient to move, symptom reproduction, the pattern and range of movement and muscle control. The range of movement can be measured using a goniometer or visual estimation. When following patients with haemophilic arthropathy over time, a progressive loss of range of movement may be apparent [17].

If active movements are symptom-free, overpressure can be applied with care to test the end-feel [7]. The joint is considered to be normal if there is pain free, full range of movement and the end-feel is normal [7]. Joints above and below the area of symptoms can be tested using clearing movements.

Passive physiological movements. During passive movements the joint is moved by the physiotherapist. The physiotherapist will be feeling for the quality of the available range, detecting instances of hypermobility, i.e. excessive range of movement or hypomobility, as indicated by reduced range or increased resistance. The physiotherapist should establish the quality of the end-feel for each movement, i.e. bony or soft tissue end-feel. In patients with arthropathy associated with contractures, a soft tissue end-feel indicates that physiotherapy may be able to improve range of movement. A bony, hard end-feel will be less responsive to manual techniques.

Passive accessory movements. Accessory movements are the sliding movements which occur between articular surfaces and are a normal part of physiological movement. If testing active or passive physiological movement has reproduced pain and/or is limited by resistance then accessory movements can be tested [3]. Accessory movements can be used to identify and localize the symptomatic joint, to define the nature of joint motion and abnormality and provide a basis for the selection of treatment techniques [6]. The physiotherapist should feel for the quality and range of movement, pain response, resistance and muscle spasm (Fig. 1.1).

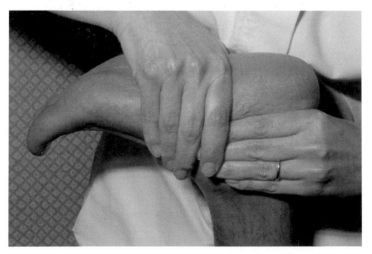

Figure 1.1 Assessment of accessory range of movement in the ankle joint.

Muscle tests

Static (isometric) voluntary muscle contraction can be assessed. The joint is placed in a neutral position and the physiotherapist applies manual resistance. The advantages of isometric testing in patients with haemophilia is that the muscles can be assessed without moving the joint which may be painful particularly following a bleed or in cases of arthropathy. Marked muscle weakness may be apparent as a result of pain and inhibition of muscles and disuse. The degree of muscle atrophy can be estimated by measuring limb circumference with a tape measure. The physiotherapist may also wish to test manual resistance through range, i.e. isotonic power if the joint movement is not painful.

Muscle imbalance. Recently a great deal of research has focused on the correct activation and co-ordinated timing of muscle action [18]. Muscle balance is defined as the balance between different muscle groups so that there is the correct loading and alignment of the joints. Muscles with a predominately mobilizing role, for example hamstrings, tensor tascia lata or gastrocnemius, may become tight and overactive. These muscles are assessed for appropriate length. Muscles with a predominately stabilizing role (e.g. gluteals, lower fibres of trapezius or transversus abdominis) often become inhibited in the presence of pain and are assessed by testing their endurance capacity and ability to hold in inner range positions [18]. Muscle imbalance has been described in patients with haemophilia either associated with bleeds in muscles or joints or as a result of synovitis or arthropathy [19]. For example, gastrocnemius is a common site of bleeding and may become shortened and overactive. This can influence both ankle and knee positions, leading to altered biomechanics at these joints and others within the lower limb kinetic chain. Muscle imbalance can also occur around the knee. Weakness of vastus medialis oblique and overactivity of vastus lateralis and other lateral structures can cause patella maltracking and anterior knee pain. The static and dynamic position of the patella can be assessed [20] (Fig. 1.2).

Neurological examination

In patients with haemophilia peripheral neuropathies may be

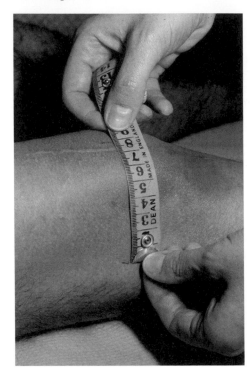

Figure 1.2 Assessing static lateral glide of the patella.

associated with bleeds and therefore the neurological system must be assessed if the patient complains of neurological symptoms. This includes testing cutaneous sensibility, muscle power and tendon reflexes. Femoral nerve neuropathy may be associated with iliopsoas bleeds causing quadriceps weakness (which may be marked) and sensory loss over the anterior aspect of the thigh. Elbow bleeds may cause neuropathies of the ulnar nerve with sensory loss over the ulnar aspect of the forearm and hand, and weakness of the interossei.

Specific neural tissue tension tests, e.g. Straight Leg Raise or Upper Limb Tension Tests [21] can be used with care in haemophilic patients to assess the mobility of the nervous system. For example, careful assessment of nervous tissue mobility by Upper Limb Tension Test 3 may be indicated in patients with mild sensory symptoms in the ulnar nerve distribution. The physiotherapist will assess the range, quality, pain and resistance. A positive response is indicated by the reproduction of the patients symptoms, production of a response different to an expected normal response or reduced range of movement compared to the other limb.

Other tests

Specific regional examinations may include additional tests. For example examination of the knee should include careful passive examination of the cruciate and collateral ligaments because laxity may occur secondary to bleeds in the absence of other trauma.

Bleeds in children may lead to hyperaemia at the epiphyseal plates with resultant bone overgrowth [1]. In the lower limb this can result in true leg length differences, therefore leg length should be measured. This abnormality can be associated with a flexion deformity of the knee and can also lead to increased stress on other joints.

Specific proprioception and balance assessment can also be performed, particularly in patients with chronic synovitis or arthropathy of the lower limb joints [22].

Palpation

The patient should be supported in a comfortable position for palpation. Increased temperature, swelling and tenderness may be associated with an acute bleed. If the patient has swelling, the physiotherapist should establish whether this is primarily due to a fluid within the joint or a more 'boggy' feel due to thickened synovium. In cases of advanced arthropathy, bony changes may be palpable and even emphasized by the concomitant loss in muscle bulk.

Recording and planning treatment

Systematic recording will assist the physiotherapist in their reasoning process and in planning the patient's management. Problem orientated medical records (POMR) encourages the physiotherapist to identify problems from the patient's perspective. From this problem list, goals for treatment can be negotiated with the patient [23]. Goals should be SMART, i.e. specific, measurable, attainable, realistic and timebased. It is important to consider an individual's predisposition to bleeding and stage of arthropathy when determining the goals.

Conclusion

The key to successful management is a thorough and detailed assessment. Treatment is tailored to the individual based on the examination findings. Reassessment of both subjective and physical examination markers and clear goal setting will enable the interventions to be evaluated. The future for these patients is continually improving with enhanced medical and surgical management, however, patients still present with musculoskeletal dysfunction. The physiotherapist, with a wide range of assessment and management skills is in an ideal position to improve and maintain the musculoskeletal health of these patients.

References

1 Rodriguez-Merchan E.C. Effects of hemophilia on articulations of children and adults. *Clin Orthop* 1996; 328: 7–13.
2 Cahill M, Colvin B. Haemophilia. *Postgrad Med J* 1997; 73: 201–6.
3 Maitland G. *Vertebral Manipulation*, 5th edn. London: Butterworths, 1986.
4 Jones M. Clinical reasoning process in manipulative therapy. In: Boyling J, Palastanga N, eds. *Grieve's Modern Manual Therapy*, 2nd edn. Edinburgh: Churchill Livingstone, 1994: 471–89.
5 Brettler D. Inhibitors in congenital haemophilia. *Bailliere's Clinical Haematology* 1996; 9(2): 319–30.
6 Petty N, Moore A. *Neuromusculoskeletal Examination and Assessment.* Edinburgh: Churchill Livingstone, 1998.
7 Maitland G. *Peripheral Manipulation*, 3rd edn. London: Butterworth-Heinemann, 1991.
8 Murtagh J, Kenna C. *Back Pain and Spinal Manipulation*, 2nd edn. London: Butterworth-Heinemann, 1997.
9 Heim M, Horoszowski H, Seligsohn U, Martinowitz U, Strauss S. Iliopsoas hematoma — its detection and treatment with special reference to hemophilia. *Arch Orthop Trauma Surg* 1982; 99: 195–7.
10 Miller R, Beeton K, Goldman E, Ribbans W. Counselling guidelines for managing musculoskeletal problems in haemophilia in the 1990s. *Haemophilia* 1997; 3: 9–13.
11 Gilbert M, Aledort L, Seremetis S, Needleman B, Oloumi G, Forster A. Long term evaluation of septic arthritis in hemophilic patients. *Clin Orthop* 1996; 328: 54–9.
12 Gregg-Smith S, Pattison R, Dodd C, Giangrande P, Duthie R. Septic arthritis in haemophilia. *Br J Bone Joint Surg* 75-B 1993; 3: 368–70.

13 Ribbans W, Giangrande P, Beeton K. Conservative treatment of haemarthrosis for prevention of hemophilic synovitis. *Clin Orthop* 1997; 343: 12–18.

14 Jones M. Clinical reasoning in manual therapy. *Phys Ther* 1992; 72 (12): 875–84.

15 Kendal F, McCreary E, Provance P. *Muscle Testing and Function*, 4th edn. Baltimore: Williams & Wilkins, 1983.

16 Heim M, Horoszowski H, Martinowitz U. Leg-length inequality in haemophilia. *Clin Pediatr* 1985; 24(10): 601–2.

17 Johnson R, Babbitt D. Five stages of joint disintegration compared with range of motion in hemophilia. *Clin Orthop* 1985; 201: 36–42.

18 Richardson C, Jull G, Hodges P, Hides J. *Therapeutic Exercise for Spinal Segmental Stabilisation in Low Back Pain*. Edinburgh: Churchill Livingstone, 1999.

19 Beeton K, Cornwell J, Alltree J. Muscle rehabilitation in haemophilia. *Haemophilia State of the Art* 1998; 4: 532–7.

20 McConnell J. Management of patello–femoral problems. *Manual Ther* 1996; 1(2): 60–6.

21 Butler D. *Mobilisation of the Nervous System*. Edinburgh: Churchill Livingstone, 1991.

22 Buzzard B. Proprioceptive training in haemophilia. *Haemophilia State of the Art* 1998; 4(4): 528–31.

23 Cott C, Finch E. Goal setting in physical therapy practice. *Physiotherapy Canada* 1991; 43(1): 19–22.

2   Pain Mechanisms

Andrew Clements

Pain is a familiar experience to people with haemophilia. From a young age through to adulthood a person with haemophilia will experience pain. Muscle or joint bleeds, whether traumatic or spontaneous, are painful [1]. The chronic haemophilic arthropathy, so commonly seen in the older person with haemophilia, is also painful. Frequently even the treatment (therapeutic venipuncture) to prevent or minimize the effects of bleeding can cause pain. Throughout their life a person with haemophilia can expect pain. Improvements in the management of haemophilia has impacted on the previous strong link between pain and haemophilia, however, not all the people with haemophilia in the population have access to clotting factors and, in spite of these improvements pain is still experienced. Unlike other populations of patients with chronic disease processes, such as rheumatoid arthritis [2,3], pain in haemophilia has not been extensively researched but it seems accepted that pain and haemophilia are linked.

This chapter is designed to introduce current concepts and developments in the field of pain science. It is as applicable to pain within haemophilia as it is to any person with pain. The science of pain and the transmission of nociception is identical in the normal population and the population with haemophilia.

Pain as an experience

Recent developments in the understanding of physiological processes involved with pain have expanded our awareness of the experience of pain. The move away from the misconception that nociception involves 'hard wired' pain pathways is improving our understanding of pain (especially chronic pain) and hence our management of pain [4,5]. Until the past few decades, pain transmission was accepted as a hard wire system from the periphery to a pain centre within the brain. This concept was exemplified in the model by French philosopher René Descartes (1596–1650), in 'The Path of Burning Pain'. The nociceptive system is now accepted as a dynamic entity that can change its sensitivity according to the body's needs [6]. This dynamic model allows the multidimensional aspect of pain to be explored.

The current working definition of pain by the International Association for the Study of Pain (IASP) is 'pain is an unpleasant sensory or emotional experience associated with actual or potential tissue damage or described in terms of such damage' [7]. This definition acknowledges pain as a subjective experience with important affective (emotional), cognitive (thoughts), behavioural (actions) and sensory components. Pain is a bio-psychosocial experience [8]. Its multidimensional aspects will vary between individuals and will influence the actual experience of pain by an individual. The IASP definition of pain has evolved from pain as a pure sensation to a much broader encompassing statement implicating emotional factors. It also deals with actual events and potential events. Pain can be felt in the absence of tissue damage. However, it is not possible to distinguish this experience of pain from pain actually due to tissue damage. Nociceptive stimulation can lead to the perception of pain, but active emotional states influence whether and how the stimulus is perceived. Pain responses may be as much concerned with impending events as with sensation and are also influenced by prior experience and anticipation of consequence [9].

Types of pain

Three types of pain have been described: transient pain, acute pain and chronic pain. Transient pain is a pain of brief duration and little consequence. Its function is to prevent injury by initiating protective responses. Acute pain is defined as pain of recent onset and probable limited duration. It usually has an identifiable cause, either an injury or disease [10]. Acute pain is usually associated with some tissue damage and the duration of the pain relates to the healing time of the injury. Acute pain not only initiates withdrawal and escape responses, but also serves to aid the healing process by making the person experiencing the pain protective of the area. This is achieved because of the sensitivity around the area of injury to external stimuli, such as movement and touch, which could hinder the healing process [6]. Hyperalgesia and allodynia are components representing increased sensitivity of the nociceptive system at this time and serve to protect the injured area whilst the tissue repairs.

Chronic pain has many definitions. Over the recent decades chronic pain has emerged as a distinct phenomenon in comparison with acute pain [7]. For many years chronic pain has been recognized as that pain which persists past the normal time of healing. In real terms this may be less than one or, more often, more than six months. Many clinicians frequently use this chronological method, using six months as the indicator between acute and chronic pain [7], however, a definition related to the time frame is not sufficient. With many syndromes labelled as chronic pain, normal healing has not occurred within this distinct time period. It is better to consider chronic pain as that pain which persists past the time of healing of an injury when there may be no clearly identifiable cause [10]. Chronic haemophilic arthropathy, like rheumatoid arthritis, falls within this example where pain can be experienced for a long time, however, normal healing may not have occurred, hence the definition of chronic pain may be misleading in these cases [11].

Our increased knowledge about the plasticity of the central nervous system [12] in response to injury indicates that changes within the central nervous system may prolong or maintain pain for a long time after the usual time of response to acute injuries. Like acute pain, chronic pain exhibits hyperalgesia and allodynia and also exhibits spontaneous pain. However, unlike acute pain, the aetiology and pathophysiology is harder to identify. Therapeutically, chronic pain can exist due to a dysfunctional nociceptive system rather than continuing tissue damage [13].

Anatomical components of pain transmission systems

The neural circuits that are responsible for pain and the reactions to pain have been termed, 'The Pain System' [14]. Starting in the periphery, the pain system has a set of peripheral receptive elements, called nociceptors. They transmit information about noxious events to second order neurones, either in the spinal cord or brain stem (nociceptors have their cell bodies in the dorsal root or cranial nerve ganglia). At the spinal level there are interneuronal circuits that have both excitatory and inhibitory connections that interact with the nociceptive information at this level. The nociceptive signals are then transmitted to all levels of the brain by projection neurones. Further processing of the information occurs in many structures within the brain leading to the perception of pain, as well as a variety of pain reactions including emotions, reflexes, endocrine actions, learning and memory. In addition to these reactions, the areas of the brain that receive the nociceptive information can also provide excitatory or inhibitory feedback that either reduces or increases the pain response. The inhibitory feedback is mediated by descending pathways that are often called the endogenous analgesia system. There are also pathways responsible for accentuation of the pain and the pain reponses and this has been referred to as central sensitization and involves multiple levels of the pain system [15].

Nociceptors

Nociceptors are sensory receptors which detect noxious stimuli in the periphery and transmit afferent information into the central nervous system. Although often called pain receptors, this is not completely correct since it is possible to stimulate them without the person actually experiencing pain. There are many examples in the literature of serious injuries, where the person suffering the injury does not feel any pain at the time [16].

Nociceptors are activated by tissue damage, although it is the brain that processes any incoming noxious information to produce the experience of pain [6]. Nociceptors respond to three types of stimuli, mechanical, thermal and chemical and this nociceptive information is transmitted to the central nervous system by two primary afferent neurones, the small myelinated A delta fibres and the slow, nonmyelinated C fibres. Nociceptors may respond to one form of stimulus or may be polymodal and respond to all three [17]. The A delta nociceptors respond to noxious thermal and/or mechanical stimuli and are often called high threshold since they respond to high intensity input. They respond maximally to high intensity mechanical stimulation and produce a sharp, pricking sensation [18]. This is often called fast pain since the small myelinated fibres relay action potentials into the central nervous system at a speed of 20–30 m per second. The C polymodal nociceptors relay noxious information via the slow unmyelinated C fibres at conduction speeds of less than 2.5 m per second. They cause sensations often described as dull and aching. The C polymodal nociceptors are particularly sensitive to endogenous algesic chemicals released from damaged cells [6]. These include potassium, serotonin (5-HT), bradykinin and substance P. The primary afferent C fibres are far more numerous than the myelinated primary afferents.

The primary neurotransmitter substance in the primary afferent nociceptors is glutamate and its action is modulated by neuropeptides, such as calcitonin gene related peptide (CGRP), substance P, neurokinin A and somatostatin. The largest primary afferents, the A beta fibres, are responsive to low intensity stimuli (and therefore called low threshold). They are responsive to non-noxious, mechanical and tactile sensations, such as light touch, pressure and proprioception. Their impulses are transmitted very quickly between 30 and 100 m per second to the central nervous system and although they do not transmit noxious information, they do have an important part to play in relation to pain, which will be discussed later.

Additionally, it is important to mention the so called silent nociceptors [19]. Healthy, articular tissue contains nociceptors whose threshold is so high that they cannot be excited by even very strong noxious mechanical stimuli [21]. These have been called silent or sleeping nociceptors and can undergo a process called peripheral sensitization. This process (which can take several hours) results in them becoming highly responsive to even weak mechanical stimuli [20]. Peripheral sensitization is often associated with tissue injury and inflammation and results from the exposure of the nociceptor endings to inflammatory reagents such as prostaglandins, bradykinin, histamine, cytokinins and interlukins. The result is that weak, previously nonnoxious stimuli now activate nociceptors and cause pain. The tenderness of peripheral sensitization is induced by the inflammatory mediators which are also responsible for the other signs of inflammation [22].

Spinal cord level

Signals from the nociceptors are then relayed up through at least one spinal neurone prior to transmission to the higher brain regions [15]. Noxious input from the periphery is received within the dorsal horn of the spinal cord which contains both local interneurones and projection neurones to relay information about the noxious information to the higher processing areas in the brain. The afferent fibres enter the spinal cord and primarily innervate regions of the spinal cord within the spinal segment matching that spinal nerve. However, the fine afferent fibres may ascend or descend through Lissauers track and it has been shown that the primary afferents can innervate up to 6 spinal levels above and below their level of entry [15,23]. Within the dorsal horn the nociceptive neurones are generally classified as either nociceptive specific (NS) or wide dynamic range (WDR) neurones, based on their responses to mechanical stimulation of the skin [24,25]. Nociceptive specific cells are mainly found in the laminar, one of the dorsal horns of the spinal cord, and only respond to noxious stimulation. When activated they rapidly transmit information up to the brain, usually by the spinothalamic tract. The wide dynamic range neurones respond best to noxious stimuli, but they are also excited by activation of sensitive mechanoreceptors and hence get input from A delta and C fibres and also non-noxious input from the large diameter A beta fibres. Nociceptive input from the periphery may also be modulated at spinal level by either excitatory or inhibitory local interneurones and also via descending influences at the level of the spinal cord.

Central ascending pathways

Nociceptive neurones in the spinal cord have projections to many sensory processing areas within the brain, including the thalamus, the dorsal column nuclei, the reticular formation, the parabrachial nucleus, the periaqueductal grey, anterior pretectal nucleus and the hypothalamus [15]. The main pathways are:

Spinothalamic tract

This is a direct nociceptive pathway that ascends in the white matter of the spinal cord to different areas within the thalamus and the brain. From here it is projected onward to the somatosensory cortex of the cerebrum where the sensory aspects of the pain are processed. This includes information about the intensity, quality and location of the noxious stimuli [6].

Postsynaptic dorsal column pathway

The spinothalamic tract cells relay nociceptive information from the skin and other somatic structures, whereas visceral nociceptive information is passed up through the dorsal column to the thalamus via the postsynaptic dorsal column neurones.

Spinoreticular system

Many of the projections from the spinal cord innervate other regions of the brain involved in pain related activities, such as autonomic responsiveness (e.g. increased blood pressure or irregular breathing), the affective or emotional responses to pain (the depressed mood and unpleasant feelings) and the cognitive responses to pain (the meaning of the pain). The spinoreticular system is the collective name for all these [6,24,25]. Included within the spinoreticular pathways are the spinohypothalamic pathways which involve the affective components of pain transmission through connections within the thalamus and other parts of the limbic system.

Processing of noxious information at the higher cerebral cortex level remains a controversial area, although recent studies using positron emission tomography (PET) and functional magnetic resonant imaging (fMRI) have allowed for some mapping of areas of increased blood flow indicating both areas of increased activity [26,27], and areas previously not considered in the experience of pain.

The central mechanisms

Following peripheral nociceptive stimuli changes occur within the central nervous system. The central nervous system is able to alter its sensitivity quickly and easily following nociceptive input from tissue damage or peripheral nerve injury [28]. The increased impulses from all of the sensory afferents (often called the afferent barrage) alters the sensitivity state of the dorsal horn cells, which then transmit to the higher brain centres. The interneurones within the dorsal horn have their sensitivity electrochemically altered and this can cause four effects [13]. These four effects occur normally and are protective measures that allow healing to occur. However, if they continue after the time of normal healing, they may become maladaptive and create pain problems that are difficult to treat and can prevent adequate functional rehabilitation.

The dorsal horn second order cells alter their responsivity. Dorsal horn neurones that previously responded only to nociceptive stimulation start to respond to inputs from other fibres, such as the A beta light touch fibres. In this situation, normally non-noxious stimuli (light touch or joint movement) are sent to areas within the brain as a pain sensation. The term allodynia is used to describe this pain.

Dorsal horn cells enhance their responsivity to nociceptors. The dorsal horn cells are susceptible to a phenomenon known as wind-up. Following prolonged nociceptive stimulation from the periphery, cells within the dorsal horn fire more frequently and build up their frequency. They also continue to fire after the peripheral stimulus is stopped.

Dorsal horn cells increase their receptive fields. Due to the effects of peripheral sensitization and the afferent barrage following injury, subthreshold or sleeping connections can become active within the dorsal horn and then hence their receptive field increases in size.

Due to the effects of peripheral and central sensitization, dorsal horn cells may become spontaneously active. The situation can then occur where pain is perceived when there is no nociceptive stimulus in the periphery. Spontaneously active dorsal horn cells are thought to be involved with the concept of pain memory [28,29].

The four previous examples show how the central nervous system can become sensitized. They can cause allodynia, which is a pain response to a non-painful stimuli, and hyperalgesia, which is an increased pain response to a normally painful stimulus. However, importantly, it must be noted that these mechanisms can also be suppressed, both at spinal level and from higher centres. The gate control theory is an example of pain modulation at spinal level [30]. Many of the physiotherapeutic modalities aimed at pain control are thought to work through the pain gate mechanism. Nociceptive dorsal horn cells can be inhibited by weak stimuli via the A beta fibres by either touch or electrical stimulation, such as with transcutaneous electrical nerve stimulation (TENS). Additionally, stronger stimulation of the A delta fibres can also have an in-hibitory effect via descending mechanisms within the dorsal horn. It is thought that this system works through the initiation of the release of inhibitory neurotransmitters by interneurones within the dorsal horn and these switch off activity within the nociceptive transmission cells (the WDR and NS). This has the affect of reducing the amount of noxious information reaching the brain and hence reducing the experience of pain [6].

Biopsychosocial model of pain

Previously pain has been described as a multidimensional experience. The term biopsychosocial has evolved to recognize not only the biological, but also the cognitive, emotional, behavioural and environmental factors. It is important to consider pain not only through its sensory dimension (the physiology of which has been previously discussed in detail), but also the cognitive dimension which recognizes that pain alters our thoughts and the affective dimension [31]. The development of chronic pain and chronic pain syndromes are more influenced by the psychological and social factors rather than ongoing organic pathology. Treatment strategies belong in the cognitive behaviour field, rather than trying to prevent or modify the pain from the periphery.

A detailed discussion of the cognitive behavioural interventions for chronic pain are beyond the scope of this chapter. However, the importance of the biopsychosocial element must not be under estimated. Interestingly, people with haemophilia are often described as having chronic pain. However, in the true nature of the pathology, often they have recurrent episodes of acute pain and are managed thus. It is the author's experience that a person with haemophilia who has chronic haemophilic arthropathy does not develop the chronic pain syndromes seen in the normal population suffering from chronic musculoskeletal pain. This is an area that has not been specifically researched, neither have the coping mechanisms that people with haemophilia may use to deal with their pain [1].

References

1   Heijnen L. Pain control and rehabilitation. In: Heijnen L. ed. *Recent Advances in Rehabilitation in Haemophilia.* pp 54–62. Hove: Medical Education Network.

2   Watkins K, Shifren K, Park D, Morrell R. Age, pain and coping with rheumatoid arthritis. *Pain* 1995; 82: 217–28.

3   Buckelew B, Parker J. Coping with arthritis pain; a review of the literature. *Arthritis Care Research* 1989; 2: 136–45.

4   Wall P. Overview of pain and its mechanisms. In: Shacklock M. ed. *Moving in on Pain.* Australia: Butterworth-Heinemann, 1995: 13.

5   Mendelson G. Psychological and psychiatric aspects of pain. In: Shacklock M. ed. *Moving in on Pain.* Australia: Butterworth-Heinemann, 1995: 66–8.

6   Johnson M. The physiology of the sensory dimensions of clinical pain. *Physiotherapy* 1997; 83 (10): 526–36.

7   Classification of chronic pain. In: Merskey H, Bogduk N, eds. *Description of Chronic Pain Syndromes and Definition of Pain Terms,* 2nd edn. Seattle: IASP Press, 1994: 209–10

8   Fields H. *Core Curriculum for Professional Education in Pain,* 2nd edn. Seattle: IASP Press: 1995.

9   Melzack R, Wall P. *The Challenge of Pain.* London: Penguin Books, 1988.

10 Ready L, Edwards W. *Management of Acute Pain: A Practical Guide.* Seattle: IASP Press, 1992.

11 Bonica J. *The Management of Pain.* Philadelphia: Lea & Febiger, 1953.

12 Wall P. Introduction. In: Wall P, Melzack R, eds. *The Textbook of Pain,* 3rd edn. Edinburgh: Churchill Livingstone, 1994: 3–8.

13 Woolf C. The dorsal horn: state-dependent sensory processing and the generation of pain. In: Wall P, Melzack R, eds. *The Textbook of Pain,* 3rd edn. Edinburgh: Churchill Livingstone, 1994: 101–12.

14 Willis W. *The Pain System: The Neural Basis of Nociceptive Transmission in the Mammalian Nervous System.* Basel: Karger, 1985.

15 Westlund K. Introduction to the basic science of pain and headache for the clinician: Anatomical concepts. In: Max M, ed. *Pain: An updated review.* Seattle: IASP Press, 1999: 547–59

16 Beecher H. *The Measurement of Subjective Responses.* New York, Oxford University Press: 1959.

17 Belmonte C, Cervero F, eds. *Neurobiology of Nociceptors.* Oxford: Oxford University Press, 1996.

18 Torebjork E. Nociceptive and non-nociceptive afferents contributing to pain and hyperalgesia in humans. In: Willis W, ed. *Hyperalgesia and Allodynia.* New York: Raven Press, 1992: 135–9.

19 Schmidt R, Schable H, Messlinger K, Heppelmann B, Hanesch U, Pawlak, M. Silent and active nociceptors: structure, functions and

clinical implications. In: Gebhart G, Hammond D, Jensen T, eds. *Progress in Pain Research and Management*, Vol 2. Seattle: IASP Press, 1994: 213–50.

20 Wilcox G. Pharmacology of pain and analgesia. In: Max M, ed. *Pain: An updated review*. Seattle: IASP Press, 1999: 573–91

21 McMahon S, Koltzenburg M. The changing role of primary afferent neurones in pain. *Pain* 1990; 43: 269–72.

22 Devor M. Pain mechanisms and pain syndromes. In: Campbell J, ed. *Pain: An updated review*. Seattle: IASP Press, 1996: 103–12.

23 Chung K, Lee W, Carlton S. The effects of dorsal rhizotomy and spinal cord isolation on calcitonin gene related peptide containing terminals in the rat lumber dorsal horn. *Neuroscience Letters* 1988; 90: 27–32.

24 Willis W, Coggeshall R. *Sensory Mechanisms of the Spinal Cord*, 2nd edn. New York: Plenum Press, 1991.

25 Willis W. Introduction to the basic science of pain and headache for the clinician: Physiological concepts. In: Max M, ed. *Pain: An updated review*. Seattle: IASP Press, 1999: 561–72

26 Svensson P, Minoshima S, Beydoun A, Morrow T, Casey K. Cerebral processing of acute skin and muscle pain in humans. *J Neurophysiol* 1997; 78: 450–60.

27 Jones A, Brown W, Friston K, Qi L, Frackowaik B. Cortical and sub-cortical localization of response to pain in man using positron emission tomography. *Proc R Soc Biol Sci*, 1991; 244: 39–44.

28 Gifford L. The central mechanisms. In: Gifford L, ed. *Topical Issues in Pain*. Cornwall: NOI Press, 1998: 67–75.

29 Melzack R. Gate control theory. On the evolution of pain concepts. *Pain Forum* 1996; 5(2): 128–38.

30 Melzack R, Wall P. Pain mechanisms: a new thory. *Science* 1965; 150: 971–8.

31 Gifford L. The mature organism model. In: Gifford L, ed. *Topical Issues in Pain*. Cornwall: NOI Press, 1998: 45–54.

3 Hydrotherapy and its Use in Haemophilia

Rochelle Tiktinsky and Caroline Barmatz

Introduction

The word 'hydrotherapy' comes from the Greek, 'hydro' meaning water and 'therapy' meaning healing. The use of water as a therapeutic treatment modality dates back many centuries [1,2]. The physical properties of water include mass, weight, density, specific gravity, buoyancy, hydrostatic pressure, surface tension, refraction and viscosity. An understanding of these properties is important when using hydrotherapy as a treatment modality [3–7]. The temperature of the water also has an effect on the treatment of the individual. There are many opinions as to which is the most effective temperature. Some authors advocate lower ranges of 30–32°C as this temperature is said to be optimum for relaxation [8], some advocate ranges of 35–37°C [6], while others say higher temperatures are disadvantageous to the cardiovascular system and suggest ranges of 32–34°C as optimum for relaxation and physical activity [1,9]. This chapter will discuss the therapeutic effects of hydrotherapy, techniques which can be used in the hydrotherapy pool and application of hydrotherapy techniques in the management of patients with haemophilia.

Therapeutic effects of exercise in the water

The therapeutic effects of exercise in water have been documented by Skinner and Thomson [2] and Harrison [10]. The main treatment goals are: to increase muscle strength and endurance, mobilization of joints, relaxation, pain reduction, improved balance and co-ordination, and functional activity and recreation.

Techniques of exercise in water

There are a number of techniques that can be used in the water including:
• Buoyancy assisted, supported and resisted exercises;
• Bad Ragaz techniques;
• hold–relax techniques;
• rhythmic stabilization techniques;
• repeated contractions;
• breathing exercises;
• techniques using hydrodynamic principles such as buoyancy, turbulence and balance; and
• gait training.
Stretching techniques may also be included, especially for lower extremity musculature.

Buoyancy assisted, supported, and resisted exercises

Exercises are performed while the patient is lying supported on a submerged plinth, with flotation equipment, or in the sitting or standing positions while grasping the side of the pool for support [2,11]. A series of exercises can be designed from assisted movements progressing to supported and then resisted. It is important that the correct instructions are given to the patient so that the movement is performed correctly. An increased lever arm, additional floatation devices, and increased speed, range of movement and the number of repetitions all aid in the progression of the exercises [1].

Bad Ragaz techniques

Bad Ragaz patterns have their origin in Germany, but were adapted and developed in Bad Ragaz, Switzerland [12]. Bad Ragaz techniques use the properties of water while allowing for normal anatomical and physiological function of muscles and joints. Muscle groups work together in mass movement patterns around the axis of the joint.

This method is based on the premise that when a body moves through water, differences in pressure occur around that body called the bow-wave formation [2]. Pressure rises in the area that is anterior to the direction of movement. Turbulence occurs in the area of lower pressure. Varying the pressures either anteriorly or posteriorly can cause resistance to the movement. The physiotherapist acts as a fixed point around which the patient moves. The patient lies in the supine position with floatation devices around their pelvis, extremities and neck for support. The movement of the patient is towards, away or around the therapist. Different muscles of the body can be strengthened by changing the direction of movement and changing hand placements. Techniques such as successive induction, slow reversals and stabilization techniques can be used. The therapist will have more control over the movement if the manual holds are more proximal. As the patient improves, the therapist can move to a more distal hold on the patient. The patterns have been classified as isotonic and isometric [2]. In the isometric patterns, the patient holds his limbs in a set pattern while being pushed through the water. An example of an isotonic pattern for the lower extremity is:

hip: extension–abduction–medial rotation;

knee: extension;

foot: plantar flexion and eversion.

The patient lies supine with floatation supports. The physiotherapist stands at the patient's feet and slightly to the side of the extremity that will be exercised. The starting position is: hip: flexion–adduction–lateral rotation; knee: flexion; and foot: dorsiflexion and inversion.

The command to the patient is to 'point toes, turn the knee in and push'. The physiotherapist is stable and guides and resists all the movements from distal to proximal so that the movement is co-ordinated and smooth. The patient relaxes at the end of the movement.

Hold-relax techniques

This method is based on maximal resistance of an isometric contraction [13]. It achieves relaxation where muscle spasm may be causing or associated with pain. There is no joint motion and there is a gentle increase in resistance applied to the limb.

Rhythmic stabilization techniques

Rhythmic stabilization employs isometric contraction of antagonist and agonist patterns which result in co-contraction [14]. It may be used at any point in the range of motion, using all or part of the range and incorporates the rotational component of the motion. It also helps to increase muscle strength, improve balance and co-ordination.

Repeated contractions

Repeated contraction is a technique of emphasis. It uses isotonic contractions following initial isometric contraction and it is a sustained and repeated effort in one direction [14]. This technique is indicated in conditions where weakness, lack of endurance and imbalance exist.

Breathing exercises

The purpose of breathing exercises are to:
- increase costal expansion;
- stimulate the intrinsic muscles of respiration and the diaphragm [14];
- increase vital capacity;
- increase range of lateral flexion and rotation to the trunk [2].

The starting position of the patient is supine using a water mat or plinth. The patient's lower extremities are moved passively to one side, producing a stretch along the opposite side of the trunk. The therapist places a hand on the lateral chest wall of the side that is stretched. Before inhalation, a slight stretch is applied to the legs and a slight stretch to the ribs in a downward and medial direction. The stretch is maintained during inspiration and slightly decreased during expiration. The patient breathes normally several times and the process is repeated. This technique can also be performed with the lower extremities rotated to one side.

Techniques using buoyancy, turbulence and balance in water

The patterns can be conducted in four main starting positions — standing, sitting, kneeling, and lying [2,11]. Some examples follow.

Placing the body into a curled or flexed position will change the centre of buoyancy. The physiotherapist, while holding the patient around the waist and around the knees, will be able to rock the patient forward and back, which will help promote flexion and extension. If rocked or tilted from side to side, cervical lateral flexion is encouraged.

Rotating the trunk causes rotation of the cervical spine. The patient lies in the supine position while the therapist rolls the patient in one direction, then the other. The patient is asked to rotate the head in the opposite direction to which the body was rolled [3].

Gait training

While teaching ambulation in the water, both turbulence and buoyancy can be used to improve strength and co-ordination. A progressive strengthening programme can include changing body position, increasing turbulence and decreasing buoyancy. The treatment plan can include weight transfers from side to side and forward and back and walking forward, backwards and sideways.

Therapeutic swimming

Therapeutic water programmes can help the patient learn the proper swimming strokes, improve cardiovascular efficiency and give the patient self confidence [7,13]. Newer techniques being used are the Halliwick method [15], Watsu [16], the Jahara technique [17] and Ai-Chi (aquatic T'ai Chi) [16].

Halliwick method

The Halliwick method is a technique that teaches swimming to handicapped children and adults, emphasizing entrance and exit into and out of the water, and changing positions in the water.

Watsu

Watsu [16] applies the moves and stretches of Zen Shiatsu. The movements create stretch and relaxation of each of the body segments. The patterns are sequenced beginning with the Basic Flow and the transitions that are needed to change position.

Jahara technique

The Jahara technique [17] is passive treatment in warm water, based on freedom with support, effortlessness, slow intensity and trust. Its principles include non-friction, up-thrust, head lead, traction, axial balance and hip-centred motion. These movements aim to lengthen and expand the vertebral column, which lowers the pressure on the nerve roots and causes a feeling of relaxation, freedom of movement and improved physical and emotional well being.

Ai Chi

Ai-Chi, is aquatic T'ai Chi [16]. It includes breathing techniques, upper limb, lower limb and total limb movements.

Treatment of the patient with haemophilia using hydrotherapy

This may include the treatment of a painful or stiff joint after a haemarthrosis, joint synovitis, chronic arthritic pain, mobilization after long periods of bed rest or after a splint is removed. The clinical signs and symptoms of bleeding can include [18]:

- pain;
- muscle spasm;
- muscle shortening;
- muscle weakness;
- limitation of movement;
- joint contractures; and
- decreased functional ability.

The aims of treatment in the water are:
- relief of pain and muscle spasm;
- restore and improve muscle strength around the affected joints;
- reduce joint contracture, help stretch the shortened muscles and increase range of motion; and
- re-educate functional ability.

Treatment techniques

Relaxation

The patient should be supported with floatation devices. Slow, rhythmical movements can help the patient feel at ease in the new environment. Breathing exercises and slow supported movement in the pool helps to reduce muscle spasm. The techniques such as Watsu and Jahara can be utilized.

Mobilization

While the patient is supported, active assisted movements can be carried out to the target joints. The Bad Ragaz techniques moving the limbs and trunk isometrically or isotonically [19] and hold–relax techniques can help improve range of motion (Fig. 3.1).

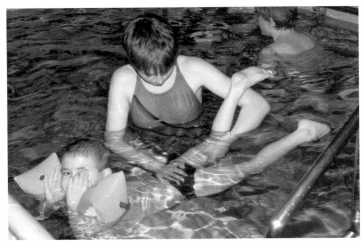

Figure 3.1 Working on hip extension in the pool.

Strengthening

Muscle strengthening can be accomplished by isometric contraction using buoyancy at first to assist, support then resist. Turbulence can be used by increasing the speed and/or changing the lever arm in order to progress (Fig. 3.2). Other techniques may be used such as contract–relax and proprioceptive neuro-

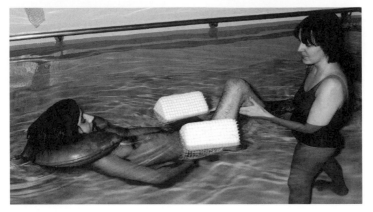

Figure 3.2 Strengthening work for the lower limb.

muscular facilitation (PNF) patterns. PNF is a technique that promotes or hastens the response of the neuromuscular mechanism through stimulation of the proprioreceptors. Patterns of movement are enhanced through normal muscular movement [14].

Ambulation

Gait training can be taught by first having the patient exercise in a sitting position. Emphasis should be placed initially on surrounding joints and later emphasis can be placed on the target joint. Foot and ankle dorsiflexion and plantarflexion and knee extension can be the first movements practised. The patient can then progress to walking in the water initially by ambulating behind the physiotherapist, so that the resistance is reduced. To increase resistance, the patient walks freely, and to continue the progression, the physiotherapist can walk behind the patient causing a drag effect.

Hydrotherapy following surgical procedures

Hydrotherapy can also be indicated following surgical procedures such as joint arthroplasty, arthroscopy, synovectomy, patellectomy, or post-fracture.

The clinical signs and symptoms experienced may include:
- pain and muscle spasm, bruising and swelling. The warmth of the water and buoyancy reduces the pain and muscle spasm and

increases circulation. At the greatest depth of the water, swelling can be reduced;

- limitation of joint movement. Mobility exercises such as hold–relax, passive movements and active assisted movements can improve limited joint motion;
- muscle weakness. Re-educating muscles using buoyancy assisted, increasing to neutral, and progressing to buoyancy resisted programmes can be incorporated. Stabilizing techniques can improve muscle balance;
- poor co-ordination and balance. Due to the buoyancy of the water, the patient will be able to stand in the water with minimal or no support. Techniques using turbulence around the patient and the use of stabilization are some of the treatment methods available.

Hydrotherapy post-knee synovectomy can be used to strengthen the quadriceps from a buoyancy assisted position and increasing to a buoyancy resisted position. Relaxation techniques can be used to relieve muscle spasm and tenderness. To improve joint motion, hold–relax and hold–contract techniques on the quadriceps and hamstrings can be implemented. Balance and co-ordination can be improved in sitting and standing using turbulence and floatation devices.

In total knee arthroplasty, knee flexion must be encouraged through relaxation exercises at first, then building up to mobility patterns and then strengthening techniques. Weight bearing, balance and co-ordination are emphasized as well. Surrounding joints should also be treated if stiffness, muscle weakness and disuse atrophy is evident.

Learning the proper swimming strokes

Swimming is one of the most positive means of activity in order to maintain mobility, cardiovascular fitness and social and psychological benefits (Fig. 3.3). Proper teaching of swimming strokes and modification for disabilities should be used [20]. Floating on the back while using floatation devices is very reassuring. Progressing to the backstroke from this position is easily done. The Australian crawl is suitable since it does not place the knee in a rotational movement during the stroke.

A method used by swimming instructors for the handicapped is the Halliwick Method [15]. All activities initially should start

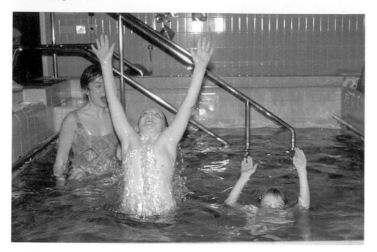

Figure 3.3 Using the water for recreation — jumping and having fun.

in a flexed position and, as balance and co-ordination are acquired, can progress to longer shapes. The exercises can be performed as follows:

1 a primary activity in which the person practices the creation of a movement or a shape;

2 a follow up activity requiring the movement of the shape to be performed against the effect of turbulence;

3 an oblique activity which can include the primary activity. The proper breathing technique is also emphasized.

Hydrotherapy and paediatrics

It is of the utmost importance that infants familiarize themselves with water. The child with haemophilia may begin to have haem-arthroses or muscle bleeds at an early age. Their movements, weight bearing, balance, co-ordination and functional activity may be impaired. The main treatment aims are to introduce the child to the water, practice breathing control, head control, symmetry and balance. If a bleeding episode has occurred recently, then the goals also include reduction of pain and muscle spasm and an increase in mobility.

The use of floatation devices is effective in order to help the child relax and gain confidence. Activities using floating toys, songs and games can be used to encourage joint movement, trunk rotation, posture improvement, balance and co-ordination.

Blowing at a floating toy in the water will help to encourage the beginnings of proper breathing control in the water.

Conclusion

In conclusion, water as a treatment environment is one of the most useful, relaxing, and variable modes of treatment. It can be used to treat a variety of situations that the patient with haemophilia will encounter and can be used to treat patients of any age. Its recreational intention can be adapted to include a clearly focused treatment plan which can be progressed. It gives the patient confidence, autonomy of movement, and eventually the independence to practice the exercises and swimming strokes at an independent level.

References

1 Reid Campion M. *Adult Hydrotherapy A Practical Approach*, 1st edn. Oxford: Heinemann Medical Books, 1990.
2 Skinner AT, Thomson AM, eds. *Duffield's Exercise in Water*, 3rd edn. London: Bailliere Tindall, 1989.
3 Reid Campion M. *Hydrotherapy in Paediatrics*. Oxford: Heinemann Medical Books, 1985.
4 Macdonald F. *Mechanics for Movement*. London: F. Bell and Sons, 1973.
5 Massey BS. *Mechanics of Fluids*, 4th edn. New York: Van Nostrand Reinhold Company, 1979.
6 Davis BC, Harrison RA. *Hydrotherapy in Practice*. Edinburgh: Churchill Livingstone, 1988.
7 Smith DW, Bierman EL, *The Biological Ages of Man — from Conception Through to Old Age*. Philadelphia: WB Saunders, 1973.
8 Vleminckx M. Pregnancy and recovery: the aquatic approach in obstetrics and gynaecology. In: Mckenna J, eds *Obstetrics and Gynaecology*. Edinburgh: Churchill Livingstone, 1988: 00–0.
9 Franchimont P, Juchmes J, Lecomte J. Hydrotherapy Mechanisms and Indications. *Pharmacol Ther* 1983; 20: 79–93.
10 Harrison RA. Hydrotherapy in rheumatic conditions. In: Hyde S A, ed. *Physiotherapy in Rheumatology*. Oxford: Blackwell Scientific Publications, 1980.
11 Bolton E, Goodwin D. *An Introduction to Pool Exercises*. Edinburgh: Churchill Livingstone, 1974.
12 .Boyle AM. The Bad Ragaz ring method. *Physiotherapy* 1981; 67: 99.
13 Knott M, Voss B, eds. *Proprioceptive Neuromuscular Facilitation-Patterns*

and *Techniques*, 2nd edn. New York: Harper & Row Publishers Medical Department, 1968.

14   Slade C, Simmons-Grab D. Therapeutic swimming as a community based program. *Cognitive Rehab* 1987; March–April: 18–20.

15   Martin J. The Halliwick method. *Physiotherapy* 1981; 67(10): 288–91.

16   Dull Harold. *WATSU Freeing the Body in Water*, 2nd edn. California: Harbin Springs Publishing, 1997.

17   Rosen, T.J. *Technique POB*. 3696 Hod Hasharon Israel: 1999.

18   Duthie RB, Rizza CR, Giangrande PLF, Dodd CAF. *The Management of Musculoskeletal Problems in Haemophilia*, 2nd edn. Oxford: Oxford University Press, 1994.

19   Davis BC. A technique of re-education in the treatment pool. *Physiotherapy* 1967; 63(2): 57–9.

20   Elkington HJ. *Swimming: A Handbook for Teachers*. Cambridge: Cambridge University Press, 1978.

4 Electrotherapy and its Use in Haemophilia

Mandy Higginbottom and Victoria Leckie

This chapter will discuss the electrotherapy modalities of pulsed short-wave diathermy (PSWD) and ultrasound (US) that are used at the Royal Hallamshire Hospital, Sheffield, in the management of bleeds and arthropathy flare-ups in patients with haemophilia. We recognize that other electrotherapy modalities are used but this chapter will focus on our preferred choice for the management of haemarthroses in these patients.

Pulsed short-wave diathermy

Pulsed short-wave diathermy is the application of separate pulses of high frequency electromagnetic energy to the tissues. The duration of each pulse is measured in microseconds and the number of pulses per second in hertz (Hz). These puls-ing parameters can be varied on most machines. Pulsing the electromagnetic energy with a short 'on' time and a prolonged 'off' time allows high levels of energy to be applied during a pulse but overall the mean power delivered to the patient is kept low [1].

There is an element of heating that occurs during the 'on' pulse, but this is dissipated during the 'off' phase. It is therefore possible to give treatment with no net increase in tissue temperature and therefore PSWD can be used safely in patients with haemophilia. The nonthermal effects of the modality are those generally considered to be therapeutically more significant.

There are two types of output from the PSWD machines, the electric field and the magnetic field. Some machines offer the ability to pulse either output, while others offer a special screen in the face of the drum which is used to generate the electromagnetic energy to eliminate the electrical field.

Effects of pulsed short-wave diathermy

PSWD has been considered to act by accelerating the tissue healing process. The effects are attributed to the electric and magnetic fields the machines produce. Most research has concentrated on the magnetic field effects with many machines now eliminating the electric field.

The primary effects of PSWD have been listed by Goldin *et al.* [2] as:

• increased number of white blood cells and fibroblasts in the wound;
• increased re-absorption of oedema;
• increased absorption of haematomas;
• reduction in the inflammatory process;
• a quicker rate of fibrin fibre orientation and deposition of collagen at an earlier stage;
• improved healing of the nervous system.

Clinical evidence

Clinical research into PSWD has been conducted since the 1970s. Due to the poor recording of treatment parameters and the variety of machines used with different outputs, it is difficult to state the preferred treatment parameters in any particular injury. Low [3] however, completed a meta-analysis of those trials that could be compared, looking for differences between the successful and unsuccessful trials. He determined that the successful trials, predominately treating acute ankle injuries, applied the PSWD via a diapulse machine at a pulse duration of 65 milliseconds repeated at 400, 500 or 600 pulses per second for an average of 60 minutes. The mean power generated during these treatments was 25–38 Watts (W).

Bricknell and Watson [4] in their study found heating occurring in the tissues at a mean power of 12 W and for safety advised keeping the mean power below 5 W. Any increase in the temperature of the tissues around a bleed site in a patient with haemophilia would cause vasodilatation and a worsening of the bleeding into the area. Physiotherapists treating these patients must therefore always consider the mean power output of the machines they are using to ensure it is below 5 W until more studies are completed.

The formula

pulse width (s) × pulse frequency (Hz) × peak output (W)

is used to calculate the mean power.

The mean power advocated by Low [3] is much higher than that recommended by the authors for patients with haemophilia. However, Low [3] concluded that the daily treatment time of 60 min was an important element. The unsuccessful studies in his meta-analysis, using lower mean powers, had only 20 min daily treatment times. Hayne [5] has advocated, on the basis of successful clinical experience, 65 milliseconds at 100–200 pulses per second and a total treatment time of 45 min per day. A lower mean power may then produce beneficial results if applied for a daily treatment time of 60 min. Tsong [6] however, has shown that cells are capable of absorbing energy but only at defined frequencies and amplitudes. Cook and Bassett [7] stated that different cells, depending on their stage of health or pathology, required specific pulsing parameters. The focus of their research was in fracture healing and has, to the authors' knowledge, not been applied to soft tissue injuries. However, Hayne [5] does recommend various settings for each stage of a soft tissue injury but, although generally accepted, clinically they have not yet been exhaustively researched.

In all the studies reviewed the duration of treatment ranged from 1 to 7 days. In this parameter, there is consensus that PSWD is of most benefit in the acute to subacute phases of an injury due to its primary effect of reducing oedema and inflammation.

Contraindications and precautions to PSWD treatment

The Chartered Society of Physiotherapists issued guidelines for the safe use of PSWD in 1994 [8]. PSWD is contraindicated in patients with metallic implants, cardiac pacemakers, impaired sensation, during pregnancy and where there is evidence of cancer.

In summary, PSWD has been advocated for resolution of oedema and the acceleration of tissue healing within the first 5 days of an injury [5]. The exact mechanisms of action and the best treatment parameters to use are not known and rigorous studies are required. There are no studies of the effectiveness of PSWD in the treatment of patients with haemophilia, however the authors have used the evidence from the above studies in their work and achieved successful results. The parameters used by the authors will be discussed with the use of a case study later in the chapter. This will allow the reader to appreciate the use and timing of not only PSWD but also its relationship with the use of US, discussed below.

Therapeutic ultrasound

Therapeutic ultrasound is a form of vibrational mechanical energy with a frequency in excess of 20 000 Hz. It is produced by the application of a high frequency alternating current to the face of a ceramic crystal. This is known as the reverse piezo electric effect. The longitudinal sonic waves cause a to and fro movement of particles, giving alternating areas of compression and refraction.

Ultrasound treatment can be applied in continuous or pulsed mode. The effect of pulsing is to decrease the energy applied to the tissues. Tissue heating depends on the rate of energy absorption, not the total energy applied, therefore, as a result of heat dissipation, pulsed treatments produce negligible heating in the tissues. The frequencies utilized by physiotherapists range from 0.75 MHz to 3 MHz, with attenuation rising with increased frequency. Intensities of up to 3 W cm^2 can be used, although intensities towards the upper end of the range are potentially damaging [9]. A couplant that provides a good match of acoustic impedance must be used to allow transmission into the tissues.

Effects of ultrasound

The result of the absorption of the ultrasound into the tissues is an oscillation of particles about their mean position. This increase in molecular vibration in the tissues can result in heat generation proportional to intensity and thermal effects can occur.

Thermal effects

If heat is not dispersed and tissue temperature is raised to 40–45°C, the thermal effects of hyperaemia will occur [10]. As a result of heating in the tissues and the associated metabolic changes, there will be an increase in blood flow, dilation of blood vessels and more rapid exchanges across capillary walls and cell membranes.

Nonthermal effects

Low levels of less than 0.3 W cm^2 can produce therapeutic bio-effects by primarily nonthermal mechanisms [11]. The nonthermal effects of ultrasound thought to be biologically important include acoustic streaming and stable cavitation, resulting in improved efficiency of metabolite transport, in-creased membrane permeability to ions and the stimulation of cell activity [9,12]. Also the longitudinal waves of compression and refraction produced can result in a form of micromassage in the tissues. Summer and Patrick [13] proposed this could potentially reduce oedema.

Healing effects

During the healing process ultrasound increases the inflammatory phase of repair [14], it appears to be pro-inflammatory. Ultrasound stimulates the mast cell and platelets to degranulate and macrophages to release several chemical mediators. This results in the stimulation of the proliferation phase, which begins approximately 3 days after injury, and hence synthesis of collagen by the fibroblasts [15]. The resultant increase in circulation and cellular activity leads to a decrease in oedema, and an acceleration of the healing process. During the remodelling phase of healing, ultrasound has been shown to increase the strength and the elasticity of scar tissue [16].

Clinical evidence

Therapeutic ultrasound has been widely used since the 1950s by physiotherapists in the treatment of a wide range of conditions. Laboratory research has demonstrated the application of ultrasound results in the promotion of cellular metabolic reactions and an increase in the visco-elastic properties of collagen. It has been clearly shown to increase the rates and strength of skin tissue healing by the mechanisms described above.

In the treatment of specific soft tissue injuries ultrasound has been used with positive results to aid resolution. Middlemast and Chatterjee [17] found ultrasound superior to thermotherapy in the treatment of acute soft tissue injuries. McDiarmid *et al.* [18] claimed ultrasound appeared to improve the rate of healing of infected sores. Success has been achieved especially in the studies involving collagenous structures. Dyson [9] demonstrated that the early stages of fracture healing could be accelerated by ultrasound.

Despite theoretical benefits and widespread use, very few well-controlled, discriminative studies have been carried out into the effectiveness of ultrasound therapy in soft tissue injuries. Holmes and Rutland [19] performed a review of the literature on the use of ultrasound with soft tissue injuries. They only found three studies without any methodological flaws and of these only one found ultrasound superior to placebo, this was in the treatment of lateral epicondylitis [20].

From the research there seems to be a lack of consensus on treatment parameters in relation to specific conditions, and how much to vary them. Physiotherapists involved in the treatment of patients with haemophilia tend to use pulsed settings at low intensities in the acute stages to avoid thermal effects. Many studies have shown increased healing rates using pulsed ultrasound [21]. As conditions become less acute higher intensities can be used, with lower pulse intervals to accelerate the healing process. The continuous mode can be used in chronic conditions, to increase flexibility and extensibility of fibrous tissue, however, in the treatment of patients with haemophilia intensities of >0.5 W cm^2 would not be recommended.

Structures within 1 cm of the skin surface tend to be considered superficial and treated with 3 MHz and deeper structures treated with lower frequencies. There are differing opinions on the duration of treatment sessions, Low and Reed [22] suggest a guide of 1–2 min for every 10 cm treated, and the smallest effective dose should always be used.

Contraindications and precautions to ultrasound

There is no evidence of direct tissue damage due to therapeutic ultrasound, but potentially a number of effects could occur due to its physiological effects [16]. To avoid these the minimal intensity and highest frequency needed to produce the desired effect should be used. The output should be pulsed as appropriate to minimize heating. The treatment head should be moved continuously in relation to the tissues and ultrasound treatment should be avoided over bony prominences. Ultrasound is contraindicated in patients with rapidly dividing tissues, circulatory problems, severely ischaemic areas, recent venous thrombus, acute infection, recent radiotherapy treatment and over the eyes.

In summary, the therapeutic effect of ultrasound most commonly utilized is its effect on tissue healing. It has been suggested that the application of ultrasound to injured tissue will increase the rate of healing and improve the quality of repair. There is good evidence of its physiological effects, however, there are few well-controlled studies into its effectiveness with specific conditions, and no evidence of its value in treating bleeds and arthropathy flare-ups in patients with haemophilia. The use of ultrasound and PSWD will now be discussed in relation to a case study, to highlight the implications for their use, and recommended parameters of these modalities in relation to the stages of the healing process.

Therapeutic use of pulsed short–wave diathermy and ultrasound in patients with haemophilia

There has been no specific research on the use of these modalities in haemophilia, however, the knowledge of their effects on the tissues and evidence from other patient groups can be used to achieve desired effects through the acute to chronic stages of a bleed.

The suggested treatment regimens of PSWD and ultrasound are based on the evidence described earlier in the chapter and will be illustrated using a patient case history. The details of the patient are given in Table 4.1.

The acute stage of the bleed

The period of 0–72 hours after a bleed (or haemophilic arthropathy flare-up) is the acute stage. The signs and symptoms at this stage are inflammation and oedema resulting in pain, heat, loss of range of movement (ROM) and decreased function. Traditionally physiotherapists have not been involved at this stage but

Table 4.1 Clinical details of patient X.

Male, 22-year-old.

Haemophilia A severe (Factor VIII level 0%) with inhibitors.

Replacement therapy: FEIBA (factor treatment throughout hospital stay).

Target joints: right knee, left elbow.

Presenting bleed: right knee, spontaneous, less than 10 hours in duration on assessment.

Assessment data: joint line measurement 43 cm (baseline measurement 36 cm).

Range of movement (ROM) fixed in 45° (baseline ROM + 10–90°).

---

our knowledge and use of electrotherapy treatment can begin to influence the healing and should be initiated as soon as possible.

The patient presented in Table 4.1 had a right knee bleed. The massive amount of swelling and inflammation were identified as the main problems from the assessment. Treatment was therefore required to reduce the oedema and decrease the inflammatory reaction without increasing heat to the area, which would potentially result in more bleeding.

PSWD has been advocated in the literature as the electrotherapy modality of choice in the acute stages of injury. This is due to its main effect of reducing oedema and stimulating early healing. The need to avoid heating in the tissues at an acute stage is achieved using a mean power of less than 3 W [4]. The patient was therefore treated using a machine with the pulsing parameters; 65 milliseconds at 200 Hz [5] producing a mean power of 2.60 W. Following Low [3], a treatment time of 60 min was used (Fig. 4.2).

This treatment regimen was used for 3 days and achieved a reduction in the joint line measurement to 41.5 cm and increased ROM to + 45–75°. The patient was now entering the subacute stage of his bleed with visible improvements already made.

The subacute stage of the bleed

The period of approximately 48 hours up to 5 days after a bleed or flare-up is the subacute stage. The signs and symptoms at this stage are similar to those of the acute phase but less severe.

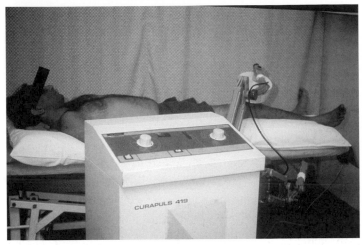

Figure 4.1 Application of PSWD to the knee.

This is when most physiotherapists treating patients with haemophilia tend to be involved, and ultrasound is often the modality of choice.

At this stage the patient's presenting problems had settled significantly. The authors hypothesize that the PSWD had helped to reduce the oedema and inflammatory reaction, and as a result the patient's knee was less painful, there was mild warmth, and 25% of normal range of movement. The emphasis of treatment at this stage was to encourage healing and repair.

Ultrasound has been proposed in the literature as pro-inflammatory in its effects, and is suggested to speed up the rate of healing and enhance the quality of repair. In the subacute phase, the aim is to accelerate the inflammatory processes, but there is still a need for negligible heating. This is achieved by using low intensities and by pulsing the source. The patient was treated using a Bosch Sonomed 4 machine. The 3 MHz head was used, at an intensity of 0.25 W cm^2 [12], pulsed in a ratio 1 : 4, for 5 min. Over the next 2 days this regimen was used with minimal reduction in joint line measurement to 41.3 cm, but ROM increasing to + 45–90°. By day 5, the patient was entering the chronic stage of his bleed, with the healing process underway.

The chronic stage of the bleed

The period 5 days after a bleed or flare-up tends to be classified as the chronic stage. The signs and symptoms tend to be related to reduced muscle strength and decreased function. At this stage the patient had some residual swelling and loss of ROM, but no signs of warmth or complaints of pain. Treatment was aimed at continuing to accelerate healing and repair processes.

Ultrasound tends to be our treatment of choice in the chronic stage of injury. This is due to its effects in the inflammatory, proliferation and remodelling phases of the healing process. At this stage higher intensities were used, with the source still pulsed in the ratio 1 : 4. The patient was treated with the same settings but the intensity was increased from $0.3\,W\,cm^2$ through to $0.8\,W\,cm^2$ with beneficial effects.

The patient was treated with ultrasound for a further 3 days, and achieved a reduction of joint line measurement to 38.0 cm and increases in ROM to + 20–95°. At this stage the patient was discharged home and continued to attend gym sessions as an outpatient to improve his quadriceps strength and physical function.

Conclusion

In musculoskeletal problems affecting patients with haemophilia, PSWD and ultrasound can bring important benefits in the overall management of the patient. Figure 4.2 summarizes the role of PSWD and ultrasound in the management of a bleed due to haemophilia, and suggests treatment parameters. PSWD tends to be used in the acute phase of a bleed, to reduce oedema and stimulate early healing. Once symptoms of oedema and inflammation begin to settle in the subacute stage, then therapeutic ultrasound can be introduced to increase the rate of healing and quality of repair.

References

1 Oliver DE. Pulsed Electro-Magnetic Energy—What is it? *Physiotherapy* 1984; 70: 458–9.
2 Goldin JH, Broadbent NRG, Nancarrow JD, Marshall T. The effects of diapulse on the healing of wounds: a double-blind randomised controlled trial in man. *Br J Plast Surg* 1981; 34: 434–9.
3 Low J. Dosage of some pulsed shortwave clinical trials. *Physiotherapy* 1995; 81: 611–16.

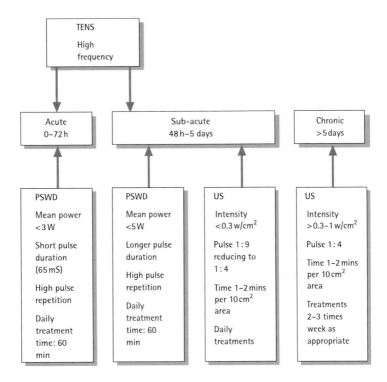

Figure 4.2 Summary of electrotherapeutic interventions following a bleed due to haemophilia.

4　Bricknell R, Watson T. The thermal effects of pulsed shortwave therapy. *Br J Ther Rehabilitation* 1995; 2(8): 430–4.

5　Hayne CR. Pulsed high frequency energy—its place in physiotherapy. *Physiotherapy* 1984; 70: 459–66.

6　Tsong TY. Deciphering the language of cells. *Trends Biol Sciences* 1989; 14: 92.

7　Cook IA, Bassett CAL. Electromagnetically-induced pulse waveforms are dependant upon tissue factors. *Transactions Bioelectric Repair Growth Society* 1983; 3: 20.

8　Docker M, Bazin S, Dyson M, Kitchen S, Low J, Simpson G. Guidelines for the safe use of pulsed shortwave therapy equipment. *Physiotherapy* 1994; 80: 233–5.

9　Dyson M. Mechanisms involved in therapeutic ultrasound. *Physiotherapy* 1987; 73: 116–20.

10　Lechmann JF, Guy AW. Ultrasonic therapy in interaction of ultrasound and biological tissues. In: Reid JM, Sikov MR, eds. *Workshop*

Proceedings. US Dept Health Education and Welfare Publications, 1972: 141–52.

11 Dyson M, Preston R, Woledge R, Kitchen S. Longwave ultrasound. *Physiotherapy* 1999; 85: 40–9.

12 Dyson M. Therapeutic applications of ultrasound. In: Nyborg WL, Zistin MC, eds. *Biological Effects of Ultrasound*. London: Churchill Livingstone, 1985.

13 Summer W, Patrick MK. *Ultrasonic Therapy A Text Book for Physiotherapists*. London: Elsevier, 1964.

14 Young SR. *The effect of therapeutic ultrasound on the biological mechanisms involved in dermal regeneration*. PhD Thesis, University of London, 1988.

15 Webster DF, Harvey W, Dyson M, Pond JB. The role of ultrasound-induced cavitation in the vitro stimulation of collagen synthesis in human fibroblasts. *Ultrasonics* 1980; 4: 343–51.

16 Dyson M. Stimulation of tissue repair by therapeutic ultrasound. In: Dineen P, Hildick-Smith G, eds. *The Surgical Wound*. Philadelphia: Lea and Febiger, 1981.

17 Middlemast SJ, Chatterjee DS. Comparison of ultrasound and thermography for soft tissue injuries. *Physiotherapy* 1978; 64: 331–2.

18 McDiarmid T, Burns PN, Lewith GT *et al*. Ultrasound in the treatment of pressure sores. *Physiotherapy* 1985; 71: 66–70.

19 Holmes MAM, Rutland JR. Clinical trials of ultrasound treatment in soft tissue injury: a review and critique. *Physiotherapy Theory and Practise* 1991; 7: 163–75.

20 Binder A, Hodge G, Greenwood AM *et al*. Is therapeutic ultrasound effective in soft tissue lesions? *BMJ* 1985; 290: 512–14.

21 Dyson M, Suckling J. Stimulation of tissue repair by ultrasound: a survey of the mechanism involved. *Physiotherapy* 1978; 64: 105–8.

22 Low JR, Reed A. *Electrotherapy Explained: Principles and Practice*, 2nd edn. Oxford: Butterworth-Heinemann, 1994.

5 Muscle Imbalance in Haemophilia

Jane Padkin

Introduction

The majority of bleeding incidences in haemophilia affect the musculoskeletal system. Muscle imbalance can occur as a result of acute bleeds, joint effusions, pain, poor proprioception, synovitis and haemophilic arthropathy. The resulting pain, swelling and tissue damage may ultimately lead to muscle imbalance and movement dysfunction. To explore this topic, current research and treatment approaches will be discussed.

In the ideal situation, the muscle system helps to minimize unwanted joint displacement and aids stress absorption, providing stability and protection to the articular structures [1]. Where muscle imbalance exists, there is inadequate control and co-ordination of muscles [2].

Muscles have three important functions. They have a role in the static control of posture and alignment of joints, a role in the dynamic control and production of movement and they also provide important proprioceptive input into the central nervous system [3].

The rehabilitation of muscle imbalance incorporates four concepts:
1 control of the neutral joint;
2 control of movement;
3 control through range;
4 regaining muscle length/extensibility [4].

These concepts aim to control pain, address the movement dysfunction and restore optimal function, thus achieving muscle balance and therefore minimizing further tissue strain and trauma in patients with haemophilia. Muscle imbalance exercises are progressed for each individual dependent on capability.

The physiotherapist introduces the exercises at the correct level following full assessment of the individual.

Kendall and McCreary [5] evaluated posture and have described different postural types. Associated with these postural types, it has been identified that muscle function under certain circumstances can change, leading to some muscles becoming inhibited, long and relatively weak and others becoming overactive, short and relatively strong. More recently Janda [3] stated that the tendency for muscles to develop inhibition or overactivity does not occur randomly, rather, typical patterns have been described. These patterns can often be seen around joints affected by haemophilic synovitis and arthropathy. Due to the alteration in normal function of the affected area, stresses may also be placed on adjacent tissues.

Classification of muscles

A major advance of our understanding of how muscles contribute to functional movement comes from recognizing their different characteristics. Muscles can be classified into two groups — stabilizers and mobilizers. They can also be further classified into local or global muscles. A useful model of functional classification has been developed describing local stabilizers, global stabilizers and global mobilizers [4].

The local stabilizers, for example, transverse abdominus and multifidus, lie close to the joints and are specialized for joint protection at a local level. The role of these stabilizers is primarily linked to joint support rather than joint movement and they seem to be most affected by injury to a region [6]. Inhibition of the local stabilizers may occur following haemophilic bleeds, due to pain, or in association with synovitis or arthropathy. Local stabilizers have an important postural and supportive role, providing stabilization of joints and therefore protection from injury [7]. They are anatomically closely related to joints. They are usually deep and act over one joint, so providing control of individual motion segments. They act continuously during activity sustaining relatively low force contractions independent of the direction of movement [8]. Research by Hodges and Richardson [9] has suggested that transverse abdominus and multifidus may be activated prior to limb movement occurring, highlighting that their role is to stabilize the trunk and provide a stable base from which appendicular movement occurs [8,9,10].

Global stabilizers provide stability and also produce movement. They contribute to the control of joint rotation. Their activity is non-continuous and is direction dependent. Muscles that fall into this category include gluteus medius, serratus anterior, the lower fibres of trapezius and the oblique abdominal muscles.

The local and global stabilizers have predominately slow twitch type 1 fibres. Muscle inhibition has been seen to occur in patients with spinal pain and the muscle fibre type has been shown to change [6]. Predominately slow twitch fibres change to type 2 fast twitch fibres. Fast twitch fibres fatigue rapidly with movement and the resulting muscle function fails to offer joint support. It is possible that muscle inhibition of the local stabilizers occurs in the haemophilic patient as a result of pain which may contribute to joint instability.

As these changes may not reverse spontaneously, even with the cessation of pain [6], it is important to restore the correct function of these muscles. Rehabilitation must begin at relatively low levels of activation of the local stabilizers [6]. Emphasis is placed on a motor skill that has to be re-learned, practised and then gradually incorporated back into functional movement [6].

Global mobilizers are more superficial than the stabilizers and often cross more than one joint, for example, the hamstrings and gastrocnemius muscles. They are capable of generating large forces and are responsible for acceleration of movement and power activities. Overactivity of the global mobilizers may occur when the stabilizers are inhibited. In this situation, the mobilizers attempt to act as stabilizers and they become overactive, short and tight, due to inappropriate recruitment. The muscle shortening may limit physiological and accessory joint motion, thereby affecting joint alignment and contributing to ongoing pathology. Overactivity may also be due to reflex spasm and pain. Trigger points may then develop within the muscle. An active trigger point usually produces a referred pain typical of that muscle, restricted range of motion and a visible or palpable local twitch response during mechanical stimulation [11]. For example, in patients with haemophilia following a shoulder bleed, pain inhibition may prevent the lower trapezius from functioning and this may result in relative overactivity of muscles such as levator scapulae and the pectoralis major and minor. Trigger points may develop in the overactive muscles, generating further pain and leading to a loss of muscle flexibility and subsequently influencing joint range.

Other factors influencing the development of muscle imbalance in patients with haemophilia

Effusions, haemophilic arthropathy, poor proprioception and pain are all factors that can contribute to the development of muscle imbalances in patients with haemophilia.

The effect of effusions

Joint effusion has been shown to contribute to muscle inhibition. The vastus medialis oblique can be inhibited by a 20–30 mL effusion, whilst the rectus femoris and vastus lateralis have been shown to be inhibited with larger effusions of 50–60 mL [12]. Hypertrophy of synovial tissue and synovial effusion, which can occur in patients with haemophilia due to repeated bleeds, may result in similar muscle inhibition [13]. The muscle inhibition may prevent the correct vastus medialis oblique and vastus lateralis ratio when performing a quadriceps contraction [14].

The effect of haemophilic arthropathy

Haemophilic arthropathy appears to be initiated by degenerative cartilage changes as a result of exposure to blood, following synovitis [15]. The articular cartilage in haemophilic arthropathy exhibits characteristics of the degenerative joint disease, osteoarthritis, whereas the synovium in haemophilic arthropathy has been shown to exhibit the characteristics of the inflammatory joint disease, rheumatoid arthritis [15].

In early osteoarthritis of the knee, muscle inhibition has been found to result in quadriceps weakness [16]. The muscle weakness contributes markedly to disability and probably renders the joint vulnerable to further damage [17] and may predispose the joint to further degenerative changes [14,18].

The following illustration shows the importance of implementing muscle balance strategies early in a patient's rehabilitation programme to minimize the joint instability that precedes further degenerative changes (Fig. 5.1).

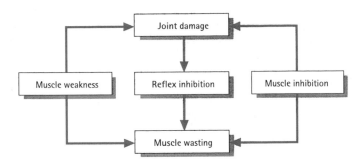

Figure 5.1 Illustration of the cycle that may occur leading to joint instability [17]. Reproduced with permission from Stokes M, Young A. *Clin Sci* 1984; 67: 7–14. (The Biochemical Society and the Medical Research Society.)

Periods of rest and immobilization following a joint bleed can lead to adaptive changes in muscle tissue [19]. These changes may influence the strength of the muscle. It is important to maintain muscle length during periods of rest and to strengthen the local stability muscles aiming to prevent muscle weakness that may contribute to further joint damage.

Proprioceptive deficits and the effect on muscle inhibition

Proprioception is defined as the ability to detect motion in joints and muscles in order to make postural adjustments to movement perturbations [20]. In healthy joints, a conscious sense of passive joint motion is in part attributed to the type 2 mechanoreceptors embedded in the capsular and adipose structures of the joint complex [21]. Type 2 mechanoreceptors are described as low threshold, rapidly adapting sensory fibres that normally fire secondary to change in mechanical stress. This may be caused by the initiation or cessation of joint movement [22]. Loss of function of these mechanoreceptors may lead to diminished awareness of passive movement. This in turn may be responsible for documented delays in muscular reflex activity around the joint [21]. A reduction in muscle activity may therefore reduce joint protection and joint support, increasing the risk of further damage. Patients with osteoarthritis of the knee have been shown to have reduced proprioception [22] and a similar mechanism may occur in patients with haemophilic arthropathy.

Haemophilic joint effusions may also affect feedback from the type 2 mechanoreceptors, resulting in a proprioceptive deficit. Chronic effusion may contribute to the inability to provide neuromuscular control and therefore lead to an increased risk of injury resulting in further joint degeneration. Guido *et al.* [23] have presented a case study describing how a knee effusion was associated with reduced proprioception.

Muscle imbalance re-education aims to improve functional performance and ideally should be combined with programmes to enhance proprioception. Buzzard describes a series of lower limb proprioceptive exercises for the haemophilic population [24]. By improving proprioception, these programmes facilitate appropriate joint positioning and muscle function and should be incorporated into the muscle imbalance approach.

The application of the muscle imbalance concept

Sahrmann [25], emphasized the importance of initially performing an assessment which identified all the muscle imbalances of the affected area, establishing the relevant diagnosis and then carefully constructing an exercise programme to address each problem. Rehabilitation takes place in stages. Initially, through formal motor skill training, followed by a gradual incorporation of skills into light functional tasks, progressing to advanced ballistic movement [26]. Beeton *et al.* [27] have used case studies to describe the assessment and treatment of specific muscle imbalance problems in the treatment of anterior knee pain and hip pain in patients with haemophilia.

To achieve optimum muscle balance, a progressive VII stage rehabilitation programme can be used [26]. The exercises address the local and global stabilizers and the global mobilizers. To facilitate this process, muscle tissue may also be treated directly through the application of trigger point therapy [28].

Priorities I – IV of the VII stage programme improve joint stability and enable good functional movement. Priorities V – VII provide dynamic stability and muscle balance for sport and ballistic movement [26]. Fast ballistic exercise should be avoided during the early training periods [6]. It is often inappropriate to progress people with severe haemophilia and joint arthropathy through to the final stages of rehabilitation. With clinical reasoning [29], the correct level of muscle training is developed for the individual. Factor levels should be taken into consideration and factor replacement should be given prior to physiotherapy where necessary. The exercises should be pain-free and should not aggravate existing joint problems.

The VII stages of rehabilitation should include [26]:

Priority I: control joint neutral with activation of local stabilizers;

Priority II: regain dynamic control;

Priority III: functionally shorten global stability muscles;

Priority IV: lengthen global mobility muscles;

Priority V: stability with added load;

Priority VI: stability with slow trunk/girdle movements;

Priority VII: stability with high speed limb and trunk movements.

Priority I: control of joint neutral

The first priority is to 'set' the joint in the optimum position for the stability muscle to be activated. The muscle is contracted to 20–30% maximum voluntary contraction (MVC) to retrain the type 1 fibres. Fatigue must be avoided. The holding time is gradually increased to improve endurance, working towards achieving 10 contractions and holding for 10 s. Throughout the muscle re-education, substitution of overactive mobilizers must be avoided, and no pain should be elicited, to avoid reflex muscle inhibition.

Following a knee bleed, vastus medialis oblique may require re-education. This is best performed in standing with a small knee bend, this position encourages coactivation of the vastus medialis oblique, the adductors and the glutei.

In the upper limb, lower trapezius, middle trapezius and serratus anterior can be facilitated in the upright position, aiming to prevent over-activity of the levator scapulae or global mobility muscles [30]. Verbal cues, and when available, EMG equipment, will give accurate feedback on the activity of the stabilizing muscles. Taping techniques can be used to help facilitate correct muscle activation [31].

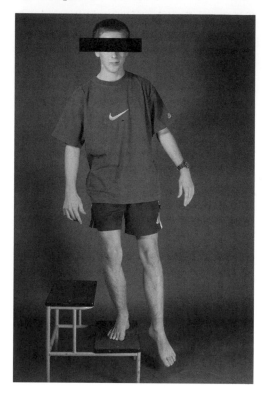

Figure 5.2 Demonstration of a dynamic knee bend in one leg stance by a patient mildly affected with haemophilia.

Priority II and III: regaining dynamic control and global stability through range

Priority II and III focus on the dynamic control of a normal movement. This will improve joint proprioception and help achieve movement control throughout range. In the knee complex the haemophilic patient may be instructed to activate vastus medialis oblique with posterior fibres of gluteus medius and then perform a small knee bend ensuring correct lower limb alignment [4]. This could be repeated 10 times progressing to dynamic knee bends in one leg stance (Fig. 5.2), stepping up and down, on and off a small block, progressing to normal step height. This use of closed chain exercise aids tonic recruitment and normal proprioceptive afferent input [31].

In the upper limb the scapula is set in the correct position using lower trapezius, middle trapezius and serratus anterior. The arm is then moved though range maintaining correct scapula control [30].

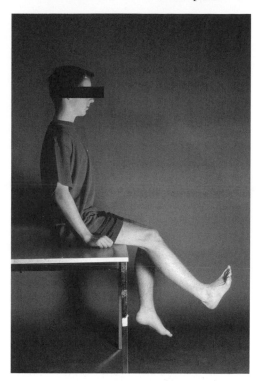

Figure 5.3 Demonstration of a hamstring muscle stretch in a patient with mild haemophilia.

Priority IV: maintaining the symmetrical length of the global mobility muscles

The aim is to regain extensibility of the global muscles that have become short and overactive. The muscles may be lengthened by using stretching techniques [3,5] and trigger point therapy [28]. Recurrent knee effusions or bleeds into the hamstrings may cause the muscle to become short, restricting hip flexion and knee extension. Contractures may then occur. The hamstring muscle length may be improved by using sustained stretch (Fig. 5.3), Proprioceptive neuromuscular facilitation (PNF) techniques or proximal active stabilizations [26]. Trigger point release work may be used to reduce muscle activity [28]. Other modalities used to treat trigger points include manual therapy, stretch and spray [28], laser, massage and exercise [32].

Acupuncture [33] or steroidal injections [34] may be considered with caution in patients with haemophilia. Factor replacement therapy may be necessary prior to the intervention.

Priority V – VII: dynamic stability for sport and ballistic movement

The majority of the haemophilic and non-haemophilic popula-tion are able to continue normal activities of daily living by achieving the first 4 levels. Some individuals will need dynamic stability for sport and ballistic movement. It is important that the control of dynamic stability has been achieved prior to progres-sing onto these stages.

Priority V: stability with added load

In level V the stability of the spine and girdles are maintained in neutral whilst resistance or load is applied through limb move-ment. The following methods may be used to achieve this. Resis-tance can be added by the use of free weights and resistance bands [26]. PNF techniques and slow reversals may also be used.

Priority VI: stability with slow trunk/girdle movement

In level VI, trunk and girdle stability is maintained during spinal and girdle movements, for example, this can be achieved by moving the upper and lower limbs whilst sitting on a balance board or a gymnastic ball. The forms of exercise that encourage level VI are Yoga, T'ai Chi and Pilates [35].

Priority VII: stability with ballistic speed and limb movement

Priority VII involves progression to ballistic movements — training stability and control under functional situations of high speed, load transition, change of direction and controlling momentum. For example, during a tennis serve it is important to achieve dynamic stability of the trunk throughout the serve, whilst ensuring stability of the shoulder complex.

Conclusion

Muscle imbalance is a developing and expanding area. It pro-vides a comprehensive approach that addresses movement dys-function in the management of the patient with haemophilia in conjunction with other techniques. From the preceding information, it is clear that muscle imbalance may occur in the patient with haemophilia due to haemarthrosis, pain, synovitis and arthropathy. The muscle imbalance approach is a flexible method of integrating muscle re-education into the management of these patients, both in the acute and chronic situation. In the acute setting, use of muscle imbalance techniques facilitates early rehabilitation and minimizes the development of dysfunction. In the chronic situation, it provides a means of re-educating movement with the aim of achieving improved muscle function and control to ensure maximum support and balance during activities.

References

1 Richardson CA, Jull GA. Muscle control-pain control. What exercises would you prescribe? *Manual Ther* 1995; 1: 2–10

2 Richardson CA. *Muscle Imbalance: Principles of Treatment and Assessment.* Department of Physiotherapy, University of Australia: Challenges, Christchurch College of Education: 1992: 127–39.

3 Janda V. An evaluation of muscular imbalance. In: Liebenson C, Butler JP, Blaker S eds. *Rehabilitation of the Spine, a Practitioner's Manual.* Baltimore: Williams & Wilkins, 1996: 97–112.

4 Comerford M. *Kinetic Control. Movement Dysfunction — Focus on Dynamic Stability and Muscle Imbalance.* Mede House, Salisbury Street, Southampton. SO15 2TZ 1999.

5 Kendall FP, Kendall McCreary Provance PG. *Muscles: Testing and Function,* 4th edn. Baltimore: Williams & Wilkins, 1993.

6 Richardson C, Jull G, Hodges H, Hides J. *Therapeutic Exercise for Spinal Segmental Stabilisation in Low Back Pain. Scientific Basis and Clinical Approach.* Edinburgh: Churchill Livingstone, 1999.

7 Hodges PW, Richardson CA. Inefficient muscular stabilisation of the lumbar spine associated with low back pain: a motor control evaluation of transversus abdominus *Spine* 1996; 21: 2640–50

8 Hodges PW, Richardson CA. Contraction of the abdominal muscles associated with movement of the lower limb. *Phys Ther* 1997; 77: 132–44.

9 Hodges PW, Richardson CA. Relationship between limb movement speed and associated contraction of the limb muscles. *Ergonomics* 1997; 40: 1220–30.

10 Hodges PW, Richardson CA. Delayed postural contraction of the transversus abdominus in low back pain associated with movement of the lower limbs. *J Spinal Disorders* 1998; 2: 46–56.

11 Hong Chang Zern. Considerations and recommendations regarding

myofascial trigger point injection. *J Musculoskeletal Pain* 1994; 2: 29–59.

12   Spencer JD. Knee joint effusion and quadriceps reflex inhibition in man. *Arch Phys Med Rehabil* 1984; 65: 171–7.

13   De Andrade J, Grant C, Dixon J. Joint distention and reflex muscle rehabilitation in the knee. *J Bone Joint Surg* 1965; 47A: 313–22.

14   McConnell J. Patellar alignment and quadriceps strength. *MTAA Conference Proceedings* 1987: 399–402.

15   Roosendaal G, Rinsom A, Vianen M, Berg M, Lafeber F, Bijlsma J. Haemophilic arthropathy compared to osteoarthritis and rheumatoid arthritis. *Proceedings of the 5th Musculoskeletal Conference*. Sydney: 1999; 13.

16   Hurley M. The influence of arthogenesis on quadriceps rehabilitation of patients with early osteoarthritis knees. *Br J Rheumatol* 1993; 32: 127–31.

17   Stokes M, Young A. The contribution of reflex inhibition to arthrogenous muscle weakness. *Clin Sci* 1984; 67: 7–14.

18   Bose K. Vastus Medialis Oblique: anatomic and physiologic study. *Orthopaedics* 1980; 3: 880–3.

19   Goldspink G. Muscle mutability; past and present research. *Abstract from Proceedings of Back to the Future Conference*. London, 1999.

20   Bernier J, Perrin DM. Effect of co-ordination training on proprioception of the functionally unstable ankle. *J Orthop Sports Phys Ther* 1998; 27(4): 264–75.

21   Lentell G. The contribution of proprioceptive deficits, muscle function and anatomic laxity to functional instability of the ankle. *J Orthop Sports Phys Ther* 1995; 21(4): 206–15.

22   Marks R. Further evidence of impaired position sense in knee osteoarthritis. *Physiotherapy Res International* 1996; 1(2): 127–36.

23   Guido J Jr, Voight ML, Blackburn TA, Kidder JD, Nord S. The effects of chronic effusion on knee joint proprioception: a case study. *J. Orthop Sports Phys Ther* 1997; 25(3): 208–12.

24   Buzzard B. Proprioceptive training in haemophilia. *Haemophilia* 1998; 4: 528–31.

25   Sahrmann SA. Posture and muscle imbalance: faulty lumbar-pelvic alignment and associated musculoskeletal pain syndromes. *Postgraduate Advances in Physical Therapy. A comprehensive Independent Learning Office Study Course*. FMI, 1987: 3–20.

26   Comerford M. Kinetic control, dynamic stability and muscle balance for sport and ballistic movement. *Movement Dysfunction Course*. Kinetic Control. Mede House, Salisbury Street, Southampton, SO15 2TZ.

27   Beeton K, Cornwell J, Alltree J. Muscle rehabilitation in haemophilia. *Haemophilia* 1998; 4: 532–7.

28   Travell JG, Simons DA. *Myofascial Pain and Dysfunction. The Trigger*

*Point Manual.Vol. 2 The Lower Extremities.*Williams & Wilkins, 1992.

29 Jones M. Clinical reasoning process in manipulative therapy. In: *Grieve's Modern Manual Therapy. The Vertebral Column* eds Boyling JD & Palastanga N, 2nd edn. Edinburgh: Churchill Livingstone, 1994: 471–482.

30 Mottram S. Dynamic stability of the scapula. *Manual Ther* 1997; 2(3): 123–31.

31 McConnell J. The management of chondromalacia patellae: a long-term solution. *Aust J Physiotherapy* 1986; 32(4): 215–23.

32 Gam A, Warming S, Larsen L *et al.* Treatment of myofascial trigger points with ultrasound combined with massage and exercise in a randomized controlled trial. *Pain* 1998; 77: 73–9.

33 Koh TC. Acupuncture therapy in haemophilia. A report of two case studies. *Am J Acupuncture*: 1981; 9(3) July–September: 269–70.

34 Hong Chong Zern. Lidocaine injection versus dry needling to myofascial trigger point. The importance of the local twitch response. *Am J Phys Med Rehab* 1944; 74: July/August 256–63.

35 Robinson L, Thomson G. *Pilates: The Way Forward.* Pan Books, 1999.

6 Exercise, Sport and Education in Haemophilia

Brenda M. Buzzard

Introduction

The benefits of exercise have been known since the earliest times. The advantages of being able to run the fastest, jump the highest and throw the furthest was obvious in order to survive. Today in the developed world, our lifestyles are almost devoid of any physical activity due to the automation and mechanization of many daily tasks. Regular physical exercise is gaining acceptance as a prescription for the prevention, management and rehabilitation of diseases. Haemophilia is a lifelong condition with a high risk towards musculoskeletal problems if not treated correctly. Physical activity, sport and sports education has been shown to reduce the consequences of intramuscular and intra-articular haemorrhages in those with haemophilia.

Benefits of exercise

It is well documented that exercise is beneficial to physical and mental well-being [1]. Most research has focused on the use of exercise as a means of prevention and treatment of coronary heart disease [2–4], asthma [5] and hypertension [6]. It is generally accepted that fit people suffer less back pain [7] and exercise can improve bone density and reduce the risk of osteoporosis in later life [8]. Exercise can improve insulin sensitivity and this may help to reduce obesity and aid weight reduction [9]. There is also documented evidence of changes in the blood clotting factors [10,11].

Physical fitness is the ability to perform daily tasks with vigour and alertness, without undue tiredness and with plenty of energy to pursue leisure activities and to cope with any unforeseen problems.

Although regular exercise may help in the prevention and treatment of certain disease processes, it also promotes a feeling of 'well-being'. Most sedentary persons who begin a programme of exercises report feeling better and have more energy within a few weeks. This effect may be psychological but physiological changes also occur.

It is important that individuals maintain an adequate range of motion in all joints. This will help to ensure optimal musculo-skeletal function. It is particularly important that individuals maintain flexibility as they age, as lack of flexibility is prevalent in older persons and is associated with reduced ability to perform activities of daily living [12]. For those with haemophilia, joint mobility and the prevention of articular or muscular contractures is paramount, and therefore promoting exercise and sport with this group of people can have profound effects on their lifestyle.

Haemophilia as a condition predisposes the person to bleeding episodes into joints and muscles which, if left untreated, can lead to impairment, handicap and disability. The stability of the joints is dependent upon strong musculature which was first described by Boone [13] in 1966. The work of Boone was the beginning of a new era in the management of haemophilia. She recognized that, instead of limiting or preventing the person with haemophilia participating in any physical activities, the opposite should be encouraged (Fig. 6.1).

Physical activity, combined with the introduction of replacement therapy using blood products, further enriched the life of the person with haemophilia. Since 1966 the literature cites many references encouraging exercise and sport as a means of prevention of articular damage. In 1996 an article by Buzzard [14], and in 1997 by Jones and Buzzard [15], carried out extensive literature reviews covering the past three decades, in which the opinions of the authors on sport and exercise were discussed. Throughout this relatively short period of time attitudes towards people with haemophilia participating in physical activity have changed dramatically. Weigel and Carlson [16] described the views of one doctor who stipulated that physical activity of any kind should be strictly forbidden. Later authors such as Dietrich [17] and Weismann [18] advised age appropriate exercise for children and modified physical education programmes.

By the mid 1990s many authors were describing more active

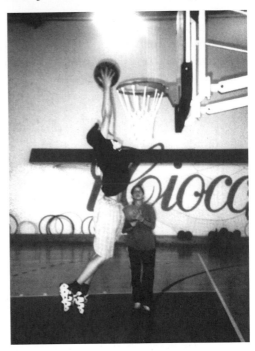

Figure 6.1 Boy with severe haemophilia playing basketball.

sports and activities for people with haemophilia. Heijnen and de Kleijn [19] and Gilbert *et al.* [20] reviewed various sports activities which also included risk/benefit ratios. Gilbert advised that contact sports such as football should be avoided.

The 1990s saw the acceptance of sport as being an integral part in the management of haemophilia, however, opinions on which activities should or should not be recommended remains controversial. In 1992, the World Federation of Hemophilia conducted a survey on sport to provide basic information in keeping with Action 1.3.8 of the Decade Plan [14,21]. In 1998 Jones, Buzzard and Heijnen [22] wrote guidelines on physical activity and sports for people with haemophilia and related disorders.

To summarize, the benefits of exercise and sport are two-fold: physiological and psychological.

Physiological benefits

- Training effect on the heart muscle.
- Decreases the viscosity of the blood.
- Increases collateral circulation.

- Maintaining muscle and joint activity.
- Control of body weight.
- Maintain lower blood pressure.
- Decrease lipids in the blood.

Psychological benefits

- Promotes feeling of well-being.
- Introduces change in lifestyle.
- Improves confidence.
- Promotes release of endorphins.
- Reduces anxiety and stress levels.

Exercise: how often and how much?

Having described the benefits of exercise and sport, the question of how often and how much needs to be addressed.

An active lifestyle protects against many illnesses and the beneficial effects are related to the intensity of physical activity. The question that is often asked is how much exercise is required to gain the protective effect. The current advice is that we should all be physically active, above our baseline activities of daily living, to an equivalent calorie intake of 1000 kCal per week, which equates to 30–40 min of moderate exercise on 5–7 days per week [23], which does not necessarily mean sporting activities. The Health Education Authority [24] recommends 30 min of moderate exercise per day as a means of promoting a healthy lifestyle. Evidence demonstrates that there is no difference between 30 min once a day or three lots of 10 min once a day [25].

The levels of physical exercise carried out by population varies between country to country and within western countries and cultures. Surveys carried out in the United Kingdom by Allied Dunbar National Fitness Survey [26] and the Northern Ireland Health and Activity Survey [27] produced the figures in Table 6.1.

Having a diagnosis of haemophilia should not exclude the person from maintaining and improving their level of fitness. Exercise and sports participation will be dependent upon various parameters such as age, severity of bleeding disorder and degree of joint arthropathy, and programmes should be adapted to take into account those considerations.

Table 6.1 Level of activity in selected populations.

	Male	Female	Min per week
Vigorously active			
England	14%	4%	20 mins × 3
Northern Ireland	21%	6%	20 mins × 3
Moderately active			
England	49%	41%	20 mins × 3
Northern Ireland	52%	46%	20 mins × 3

The use of prophylactic replacement therapy has dramatically reduced the pathological changes of the joints and muscles of those with haemophilia. However, there is increasing evidence that the level of physical activity in general is declining, and even more alarming that in children [28]. It is clear that this decline in physical fitness must be halted in order to reduce the effects of haemorrhagic episodes and its resultant sequelae. This can only be achieved by education.

Education

Education in sport and exercise is an essential component in the management of haemophilia. It should involve an holistic approach to include the person with haemophilia, their family, peers, teachers, sports coaches and friends (Fig. 6.2). Haemophilia is a life-long condition and it is important that the individual is taught from a very early age the importance of keeping active. Support and guidance is often needed for the individual in order for them to choose activities they like and enjoy, rather than being forced into doing something which offers no enjoyment.

Children, exercise and sport

The levels of activity in children have been seen to be declining over recent years and the number of obese children in the population is rising. There are a number of reasons for this increase including changes in education policies at school and changes in lifestyle.

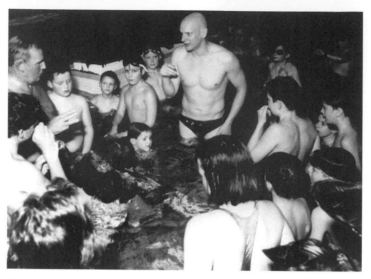

Figure 6.2 Duncan Goodhew MBE providing children with bleeding disorders advice on swimming.

Recent changes in education have moved the emphasis towards academia rather than physical fitness. There has been a marked reduction in the amount of physical education in the school curriculum. Only 30% of pupils take part in physical education at school in the United Kingdom [23]. The increase in obesity levels can also be attributed to lack of physical activity — many children are driven to school by parents rather than walking or cycling.

Changes in lifestyle, such as increased use of television and computers, have been a major influence in reducing the levels of activity amongst children. The increase in criminal attacks on children may also account for the decline in physical activity. Parents are fearful of allowing children to play outside unsupervised.

In general there is a direct link between inactivity and physical fitness. Children are now less fit than they were in the past.

For a child with haemophilia to be both inactive and obese can have a detrimental effect on their joints. They will be more susceptible to joint bleeds which, in turn, will lead to muscle wastage and de-conditioning of the supporting muscle groups.

However, at the other end of the scale there are a large

number of children and adolescents who participate in high levels of physical activity and competitive sports.

Children mature at varying rates and are structurally and physiologically different in each biological age group. Physical activities should be appropriate for the stage of physical development for each individual. When participating in team sports it is very important that children are matched for height and build rather than by chronological age.

Training programmes for children should:
- provide a positive experience in exercise for all children;
- provide exposure to sports activities and training procedures;
- aid the development of an acceptable level of health related physical fitness;
- promote acquisition of basic skills;
- provide a wide range of fitness and recreational activities;
- improve athletic performance.

The role of strength training programmes in children and adolescents has been widely debated, and recent evidence suggests that they can safely participate in properly designed and monitored programmes [29]. Jones and Mills [30] concluded, in their paper on muscle strength and training in children, that over a period of a few months there was considerable doubt as to whether weight training did anything other than train the athlete to lift weights.

The American College of Sports Medicine produced a set of guidelines for strength training in children and adolescents [31]. However it is important that anyone with haemophilia should consult with their haemophilia doctor and physiotherapist before embarking on weight training programmes, especially if they have joint problems.

Guidelines for strength training

- Physical appearance in terms of size and strength does not count—the body is still physiologically immature.
- Teach proper training techniques for all exercise movements involved in the programme.
- Stress that exercise should be performed at a controlled speed.
- Avoid ballistic movements.
- Under no circumstances should a weight be used that allows less than eight repetitions per set.

- Limit strength training sessions to twice per week.
- Perform full range, multijoint exercises.
- Do not overload the skeletal and joint structures with maximal weights.
- All strength training programmes should be closely supervised by appropriately trained people.

Sports injuries and prevention

By participating in sport one is automatically exposed to the risk of injury. Preparation is the key factor in the prevention of injuries and this preparation can often involve a collective approach. The person with haemophilia must play an active role in their own personal health and fitness to include flexibility training, endurance and strength. The instructor or trainer is responsible for teaching playing skills, gamesmanship and overall safety awareness. They are also in the position to discuss with parents, peers and the person with haemophilia potential risks and prevention strategies. It is also part of the trainer's role to make sure that the environment and equipment are safe for the purpose for which they were designed.

Parents should provide support in terms of correct nutrition and rest. Psychological support is advisable by helping the child to strike a balance between education and sport. Parental support in an active role of providing correct clothing and equipment will also reduce the risk of injury.

It is a duty of all those involved in sport and sports training to be able to identify potential risks of injury and adopt policies and strategies of prevention. This can only be achieved by education. Because children are largely dependent on adults to supervise sports activities and to act as role models, it is necessary for sports teachers, parents and health professionals to be aware of the special problems posed by children in sport.

Adults, exercise and sport

The need to exercise regularly must be maintained throughout our lifetime. Adults with haemophilia may or may not have joint arthropathy. They may also have been exposed to hepatitis B and C, and HIV. Singularly, or in combination, these conditions can have adverse effects on the person's physical ability. Buzzard [32] discussed the importance of physiotherapy and health promotion as a means of enabling the person with haemophilia to maximize their levels of independence and minimize the damage to joints caused by repetitive bleeding.

It is important that individuals maintain an adequate range of motion in all joints. This will help to ensure optimum musculoskeletal function. Participation in exercise and sport is obviously dependent upon the degree of joint damage and muscular contractures present, and equally important the level of pain experienced. Even with severe physical abnormalities some form of exercise can be performed, for example swimming is universally cited as one of the best forms of exercise for people with haemophilia [20,22]. This is because all major muscle groups of the body come into play and it also provides first class or primary aerobic activity [33].

It is up to the individual to experiment by trial and error in order to find an activity that offers enjoyment and a sense of well-being. It may be necessary to take prophylactic therapy before commencing an activity, but again each programme should be discussed with those professionals involved with haemophilia care.

The older person, exercise and sport

Due to advances in medical care and replacement therapy, the life expectancy of a person with haemophilia is the same as their peers. The body is therefore subject to the same ageing processes, namely biological, psychological and sociological. Age related biological effects gradually decrease the body's functional abilities to carry out physical activities. Biological changes occur within the cardiovascular system, pulmonary system and musculoskeletal system.

Encouragement to continue with physical activities in old age must continue. In 1994 the *British Medical Journal* stated that regular exercise increases strength, endurance and flexibility and, in percentage terms, the improvements seen in older people were similar to those in young people [34].

Programmes should include a mixture of activities tailored to individual fitness levels, tasks and interests to include swimming, walking, dancing and home exercise programmes. Older people should themselves take an active part in the planning of such activities. The general aims of fitness programmes for older people should be the same as those for younger people. Reduced joint mobility, often secondary to arthritic changes, can prove very debilitating to elderly persons. Exercise programmes should be devised to include static and dynamic flexibility in the major joints. Properly designed and graded exercises can promote the maintenance of the required levels of muscular strength. Maintaining an acceptable level of independence is often the main concern of the elderly and regular exercise can help to provide this and reduce the feeling of isolation.

Conclusion

The importance of exercise, sport and education cannot be over-emphasized, even for those who experience good health. It has also been demonstrated that exercise is of equal importance for those with chronic illnesses. Haemophilia can lead to severe haemophilic arthropathy in joints and a question often asked by patients is, 'Will exercise make my arthritis worse?'. The literature clearly shows that exercise and moderate sport can improve the symptoms of arthritis in terms of pain and joint mobility. Exercise should be within the limits allowed by patient's pain and discomfort in the affected joints.

The benefits of exercise and sport on the body system have been clearly described, and those benefits far exceed the risks as long as appropriate replacement therapy, advice and education for certain activities has been obtained.

However, of major concern is the increasing evidence of the correlation between inactivity and obesity amongst children in recent years. This is obviously a retrograde step and action must be taken to halt this process. The responsibility for this lies with us all, and education must be the focal point.

References

1 North TC, McCullagh P, Tran ZV. Effect of exercise on depression. *Exerc Sport Sci Rev* 1990; 18: 379–415.
2 Eaton CB. Relation of physical activity and cardiovascular fitness to coronary heart disease. Part II Cardiovascular fitness and the safety and efficacy of physical activity prescription. *J Am Family Prac* 1992; 5: 157–65.

3 Fentern P, Bassey J, Turnbull N. *The New Case for Exercise*. Health Education Authority Sports Council, 1988.

4 Dargie HJ, Grant S. Exercise. *BMJ* 1991; 303: 910–12.

5 Bungaard A. Asthma. *Sports Med* 1985; 2: 254–66.

6 Salomen JT, Puska F, Tuomilento J. Physical activity and risk of myocardial infarction, cerebral stroke and death. *Am J Epidemiol* 1982; 115: 526–37.

7 Frymoyer JW. Back pain and sciatica. *New Engl J Med* 1988; 318: 291–300.

8 Law MR, Wald NJ, Meade TW. Strategies for prevention of osteoporosis and hip fractures. *BMJ* 1991; 303: 453–9.

9 Blair SN. Evidence for the success of exercise in weight loss and control. *Ann Intern Med*, 1993; 119: 702–6.

10 MacAuley D, McCrum EE, Stott E *et al*. Physical activity, physical fitness, blood pressure and fibrinogen in Northern Ireland Health. *J Epidemiol Community Health* 1996; 50: 258–63.

11 Koch B, Luban NLC, Galioto FM *et al*. Changes in coagulation parameters with classic haemophilia. *Am J Hematol* 1984; 16: 227–33.

12 American College of Sports Medicine (ASCAM). *M's Guidelines for Exercise Testing and Prescription*. Baltimore: Williams & Wilkins, 1995.

13 Boone DC. Physical therapy aspects related to orthopaedic and neurological residual of bleeding. *Phys Ther* 1966; 42: 1272–81.

14 Buzzard BM. Sports and haemophilia. Antagonist or protagonist? *Clin Orthop* 1996; 328: 25–30.

15 Jones PM, Buzzard BM. Haemophilia and sport. In: Forbes CD, Aledort L, Madhock R, eds. *Haemophilia*. Chapman & Hall Publishing, 1997: 133–42.

16 Weigel N, Carlson BR. Physical activity and the haemophiliac; yes or no? *Am Corr Ther J* 1975; 29: 197–205.

17 Dietrich SL. Rehabilitation and non-surgical management of musculoskeletal problems in the haemophilic patient. *Ann NY Acad Sci* 1975; 240: 328–37.

18 Weissman J. Rehabilitation medicine and the haemophilic patient. *Mt Sinai Med* 1977; 44: 359–70.

19 Heijnen L, de Kleijn P. *Recent Advances in Rehabilitation in Haemophilia*. ISBN 0–9512694–7, Hove: England 1985: 66–72.

20 Gilbert MS, Schorr JB, Holbrook T *et al*. *Haemophilia and Sports*. New York: The American Red Cross and National Haemophilia Foundation, 1985.

21 Jones PM. *Living with Haemophilia*, 4th edn. Oxford: Oxford University Press, 1996.

22 Jones PM, Buzzard BM, Heijnen L. *Go For It*. World Federation of Hemophilia, Montreal, 1998.

23 Macauley D. *Sports Medicine; Practical Guidelines for General Practitioners*. Butterworth-Heineman, Oxford, 1999: 19–23.

24 Health Education Authority. *Getting Active, Feeling Fit.* 1996; ISBN: 0 75210510 8.

25 De Busk RF, Stenestrand U, Sheehan M, Haskell WL. Training effects of long versus short bouts of exercise in healthy subjects. *Am J Cardiology* 1990; 65: 1010–13.

26 Allied Dunbar National Fitness Survey. *Activity and Health Research,* 1992.

27 MacAuley D, McCrum FF, Stott G *et al. The Northern Ireland Health and Activity Survey Report,* Belfast: HMSO, 1994.

28 Riddoch C, Savage JM, Murphy N *et al.* Long term health implications of fitness and physical activity patterns. *Arch Dis Child* 1996; 66: 1426–33.

29 Weltman A, Janney C, Rians CB *et al.* The effects of hydraulic resistance strength training in pre-pubertal males. *Med Sci Sports Exercise* 1986; 18: 629–30.

30 Jones DA, Mills ME. Muscle strength and training. In: Maffulli N, ed. *Color Atlas: Text of Sports Medicine in Childhood and Adolescence.* Mosby Wolf, London, 1995: 101–8.

31 American College of Sports Medicine. *ACSMI Guidelines for Exercise Testing and Prescription.* Baltimore: Williams & Wilkins, 1995.

32 Buzzard BM. Physiotherapy for the prevention of articular contractures in haemophilia. *Haemophilia* 1999; 5(Suppl. 1): 10–15.

33 Weltman A, Russell RP. Principles of Training. In: Perrin D ed. *The Injured Athlete,* 3rd edn. Lippcott Raben Publications, Philadelphia, USA, 1999: 63–91.

34 Young A, Dinon S. Fitness for older people. ABC of Sports Medicine, *BMJ* 1994; 309, July: 331–4.

7 Biomechanics of the Lower Limb in Haemophilia

David Stephensen

Introduction

Haemophilia is characterized by haemarthrosis and haematomas, i.e. bleeding into joints and muscles. While most bleeding episodes are related directly to trauma it is widely accepted that bleeding is also a result of joints and soft tissue structures failing to cope with the stresses and strains placed on them [1].

Biomechanics is the study of how the musculoskeletal system responds to the loads, stresses, strains and forces applied to it during movement. When normal alignment and function of body segments exists, joints and muscles can more effectively absorb the normal stresses and strains placed on the musculoskeletal system [2]. A deviation from this normal alignment will result in more stress on the musculoskeletal system [3–5]. If the musculoskeletal structures exposed to increased or altered stress are unable to adapt then microtrauma to these tissues will result. This microtrauma in the patient with haemophilia has the potential to cause haemarthrosis and haematomas (Fig. 7.1).

With advances in factor replacement therapy people with haemophilia are becoming more active [6,7]. This increase in activity means they are placing their joints and muscles under more stress and strain. An understanding of biomechanics is thus vital for the clinician involved in treating people with haemophilia. This understanding may help the clinician identify musculoskeletal structures which are placed under increased or abnormal stress or strain and explain and prevent bleeding episodes which is the primary aim in the treatment of haemophilia.

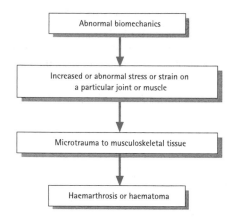

Figure 7.1
Haemarthrosis: the
result of abnormal
biomechanics.

Normal alignment

The general alignment of the lower limb can be observed in standing. This is referred to as the Q angle. The Q angle is a measure of the angle produced by a bisection of a line from the anterior superior iliac spine (ASIS) passing through the centre of the patella and a second line from the tibial tuberosity passing through the centre of the patella (Fig. 7.2). A normal Q angle would be 10–15°. An abnormal Q angle will result in abnormal loading of the patello-femoral and knee joints. Tibial rotation,

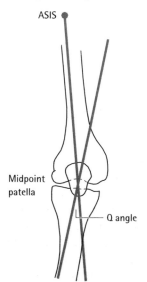

Figure 7.2 Lower limb alignment.

femoral rotation, foot pronation, leg length discrepancy and any pelvic tilt and rotation will all affect the Q angle [2,8].

Femoral rotation can be observed in sitting. The neutral position of the hip is the mid position of internal and external rotation. If there is a big difference between the range of internal and external rotation then the neutral position of the hip will be in rotation. For example, if there were 60° of internal rotation and only 10° of external rotation, the neutral position of the hip would be 25° of internal rotation.

Tibial torsion is a comparison between the axis of the knee joint and the axis of the ankle joint. The knee axis is a line bisecting the centre of the femoral condyles. The ankle axis is a line bisecting the lateral and medial malleoli of the distal tibia. It is normal to have 15–20° of lateral rotation [4]. During weight bearing there is a relationship between rotation of the lower limb and pronation and supination of the foot. An increase in medial rotation of the tibia will result in increased pronation of the subtalar joint and foot. This places the foot at a distinct disadvantage in performing its function of force absorption and propulsion during gait and alters the normal forces on the structures of the foot [9].

Normal gait

The role of the foot and the lower limb during the stance phase of gait is to:

• absorb and dissipate the compressive, shearing and rotatory forces of weight bearing;
• adapt to changes in the ground surface; and
• provide a rigid lever for propulsion [2,5,9].

Supination and pronation are the keys to the biomechanics of normal gait. Pronation and supination occur at the subtalar and midtalar joints. The function of these two joints is interrelated [10]. At heel strike the calcaneus is slightly inverted and supinated and rapidly pronates to allow force absorption and continues to pronate until the foot is in contact with the floor. According to Subotnick [10] and Donatelli [5], 6–8° of pronation is required for normal force absorption. Once in contact with the floor, the foot starts to supinate so that at mid stance the subtalar joint should be in a neutral position. Ideally, at midstance the foot should be externally rotated about 15° from the midline. As the heel leaves contact with the floor, the foot continues to supinate until toe off. According to Subotnick [10], 12° of supination is required. In total, a minimum of 18° pronation/supination is required for normal gait [5,9,10].

The ability of the subtalar joint to function as a stable joint for heel strike and propulsion and then act as a mobile joint for force dissipation and adaption to the ground is related to its function with the midtarsal joint. This is referred to as the locking/unlocking mechanism of the midtarsal joint [10]. Pronation of the subtalar joint unlocks the midtarsal joint. This unlocking allows the foot to dissipate force and adapt to the ground surface. Supination of the subtalar joint locks the midtarsal joint. This locking function increases the rigidity of the foot to facilitate propulsion.

Abnormal biomechanics

According to Tiberio [9], the presence of a deformity in the foot will result in the subtalar joint attempting to compensate for this deformity, i.e. it will alter its action or facilitate the alteration of other structures. This attempt by the subtalar joint to maintain normal biomechanics would seem ideal and beneficial. However, if this compensation becomes constant and permanent, then it becomes abnormal, thus resulting in altered stress and strain on certain joint, muscle and soft tissue structures.

If the calcaneus is over inverted at heelstrike, termed rearfoot varus, the subtalar joint would be supinated and the medial metatarsal heads would not contact the ground at midstance (Fig. 7.3). To compensate for this the subtalar joint will increase pronation and the first ray will be plantar flexed. Thus at midstance the subtalar joint will be pronated and the foot will be unstable. If adequate supination has not occurred by heel off, the midtarsal joint will be unlocked. Therefore propulsion will occur through a non-rigid foot and forces will need to be absorbed by other structures, notably the proximal joints. Increased foot pronation will produce an increase in the medial rotation forces at the knee and hip [5,9,10,11].

Increased medial rotation forces on the lower limb will produce problems at the knee as lateral rotation of the tibia is required to lock the knee into extension at push off. According to Evans [8] 40° of rotation exists in the normal knee and most of

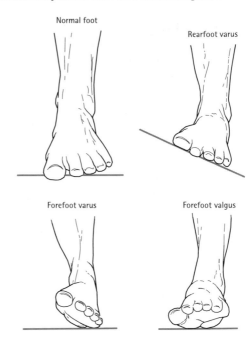

Normal foot

Rearfoot varus

Forefoot varus

Forefoot valgus

Figure 7.3 Foot deformities.

this rotation occurs in the last 15° of knee extension. This conflict for tibial rotation creates a wringing out effect on the calf [12]. This places increased strain on the gastrocnemius muscle and achilles tendon at a time when they are contracting to produce propulsion.

The subtalar joint may attempt to increase the speed of pronation immediately after heel strike to achieve a neutral foot at midstance. This will place increased stress on muscle and soft tissue structures involved in controlling this rapid movement, notably the joint capsule of the subtalar joint and the tibialis posterior muscle.

If the structural deformity in the foot is a *forefoot varus*, the calcaneus will be vertical to the ground but the medial side of the forefoot will be in varus or raised. If uncompensated, the medial side of the foot will not make ground contact (see Fig. 7.3). To compensate, the subtalar joint will pronate after foot contact instead of re-supinating. Pronation will be increased and prolonged. Depending on the severity of the deformity, the subtalar joint may remain pronated during the entire stance phase, which means the midtalar joint is never locked and stable. This greatly increases stress on other structures [5,9,10].

Another deformity of the foot is a *forefoot valgus* deformity. If uncompensated, the calcaneus will be vertical to the ground but the lateral aspect of the foot would not make contact with the ground (see Fig. 7.3). To compensate the subtalar joint supinates very early after heel strike resulting in the midtarsal joint remaining locked. The foot remains rigid and demonstrates poor adaptability to the ground surface. The forces generated by uneven surfaces will be transferred to more proximal structures.

The presence of both a *rearfoot and forefoot varus* will result in a more significant increase in subtalar joint pronation and medial rotation of the lower limb to compensate for both deformities. If the combined deformity is a rearfoot varus and a forefoot valgus proximal problems are more likely to develop. The compensation for the rearfoot varus is pronation while the compensation for forefoot valgus is supination. This provides a biomechanical conflict for the subtalar joint and problems will be transferred to more proximal structures [9].

Insufficient dorsiflexion during the stance phase of gait will produce an increase in pronation at the subtalar joint and medial rotation of the tibia [13]. The knee may also compensate by hyperextending, which will alter the weight-bearing pattern within the joint [9]. If the lack of dorsiflexion is severe and fixed, the deformity will cause a relative lengthening of the leg, which will cause a compensatory flexion at the knee or hip. This will alter the weight-bearing pattern of these joints [13].

Femoral rotation will affect the weight bearing patterns of the hip and knee and the stability function of the hip muscles. When assessing biomechanics in patients with haemophilia, the clinician must also consider the effects of pre-existing joint and muscle changes. Altered joint weight bearing patterns may be present to compensate for existing joint damage [14]. These pre-existing changes need to be carefully noted, as they will affect the biomechanics of the lower limb. For example, flexion deformities in the lower limb will automatically create a leg length discrepancy [15]. Restriction of hip rotation will result in a rotated neutral hip position. Both these faults will effect the function of the foot and subtalar joint. When attempting to correct or improve the biomechanics of the lower limb, these joint changes due to haemophilia must be considered otherwise further stress may cause further bleeding episodes.

It must be remembered that one deformity or faulty alignment can produce many compensations by the musculoskeletal system and that one compensation can be produced by many different faults or deformities. Thus determining the possible contributing factors to faulty mechanics and the extent of compensation by musculoskeletal structures is very important.

Assessment

Following a postural assessment and assessment of normal joint ranges it is necessary to find the neutral position of the subtalar joint and observe any foot deformities. To observe the neutral position of the subtalar joint, place the patient in a non-weight bearing position, preferably prone. When the subtalar joint is in the neutral position the head of the talus is equally palpable on the medial and lateral sides of the anterior ankle. The foot should be moved until this neutral position is found. At this neutral position there should be twice as much supination as pronation [5]. A line can be imagined that bisects the calcaneus with a line that bisects the distal one-third of the leg. This angle should be 0–3° inverted. An angle greater than this represents a rearfoot varus. It is extremely unusual to observe a valgus angle. If this is the case, it is important to recheck to ensure that there was no error in observation of the angle [9]. To assess for a forefoot varus or valgus the plantar surface of the calcaneus should be compared to the plantar surface of the metatarsal heads. If the surfaces are parallel then the forefoot relationship is normal. If the surfaces are not parallel the relationship is abnormal and the forefoot is in varus or valgus [9].

According to Tiberio [9], it is common for children under the age of nine to demonstrate either a rearfoot or forefoot varus due to the fact that the calcaneus and talus need to undergo de-rotation to achieve normal alignment. However if this varus is excessive it usually means that an underlying deformity does exist.

To assess leg length a measurement from the ASIS to either the medial or lateral malleolus of the ankle is taken, repeating on both the left and right sides. Using the medial or lateral malleolus will produce a different measure, so it is important to record which landmark is used.

Once any alignment faults have been detected it is necessary to see how these are compensated for by observing normal gait, or if necessary, to observe running. It is useful to use a video camera to allow closer examination. This will also be beneficial in comparing changes in gait before and after any alterations are made to correct or improve the biomechanics. Muscle length and function must also be assessed. However, it is beyond the scope of this chapter to discuss this assessment in detail. If movement around a joint is to be efficient then the correct timing and action of specific muscles is critical.

Correction of abnormal biomechanics

If any biomechanical abnormalities exist in the foot it is important to firstly differentiate between what is the primary deformity and what is the compensation pattern. This is because the underlying principle in using orthotic correction is to correct the compensation pattern not the deformity [9]. If there is more than one factor contributing to the faulty biomechanics then the clinician must identify how much each is contributing to the problem and then proceed with a correction strategy. Experience has shown that foot problems should be corrected first. This involves correcting the compensation with orthotic correction, stretches, strengthening and mobilization techniques, improving dorsi flexion range at the ankle and improving the mobility of the intertalar and metatarsal joints.

The correction of foot compensation patterns will usually require the use of orthotics, either temporary or permanent. Correction of a rearfoot varus deformity is achieved by using a medial wedge along the entire foot, stopping at the metatarsal head. If a forefoot varus exists in unison, then the wedge needs to be slightly thicker in the forefoot. To correct for a forefoot varus alone, the orthosis should consist of a medial forefoot wedge. To correct for a forefoot valgus the orthosis should consist of a lateral forefoot wedge.

It is important not to correct all of the compensation at once to avoid causing stress on other structures. The correction should be only partial initially and then more fully corrected 3–6 months later. The clinician may decide to use a temporary orthosis initially to assess the effects. Commercially available orthopaedic felt or mouldable insoles are ideal for this. The felt wedge should be placed between the insole and the shoe if possible. Corrective taping can be used initially to achieve more specific control and to assess any immediate effects.

In young children a rear foot varus is usual so if the child is experiencing no problems then no correction is necessary unless the varus is severe [9]. It is important not to correct just for the sake of correction. Following orthotic correction, the clinician needs to reassess any changes. This can be a visual alignment check in standing, video re-analysis of gait, re-measurement such as leg length or the Q angle or reassessment of pain or bleeding frequency.

In some cases, the altered biomechanics may be temporary, e.g. the result of a recent sporting injury. In this situation taping to correct the compensation to relieve stress and strain from affected structures could be considered. While correcting for foot problems it is important to emphasize that muscle weakness or tightness can also contribute to altered biomechanics and should be assessed. Muscle control should not be ignored and for the success of any biomechanical correction, muscle control needs to be normalized.

If a leg length discrepancy of more than one centimetre exists, this should be corrected. If the discrepancy is due to a flexion deformity or contracture, then attempts to reduce this deformity should be performed, if possible. If the deformity cannot be reduced or the discrepancy is due to different bone length a shoe raise in the shoe will correct the problem [16]. Femoral and tibial rotation deformities could be due to bone torsion abnormalities. If, however, it is due to soft tissue or capsular contracture or muscle weakness and tightness then this should be addressed and treated appropriately.

Surgical intervention, which is beyond the scope of this chapter may also need to be considered. The clinician needs to consider, however, how the surgical correction will alter the current biomechanics and whether the end result would be detrimental to other joints in the kinetic chain.

When dealing with already damaged joints, as is the case in haemophilia, the clinician needs to be aware that altering the biomechanics too drastically can result in transferring stress to another at-risk joint and causing joint bleeding. Gradual, partial correction is the compromise. Partial correction may not seem ideal, but it is certainly better than no correction and far better than increasing bleeding frequency in another joint and making the situation worse.

Conclusion

The primary aim in the treatment of haemophilia is firstly to prevent episodes of bleeding and secondly to prevent further deterioration in musculoskeletal structures [17]. An understanding of how the musculoskeletal system functions and responds to altered stress is essential in achieving these treatment aims. If the musculoskeletal structures exposed to increased or altered stress are unable to adapt, then microtrauma to these tissues will result. This microtrauma in the patient with haemophilia has the potential to cause haemarthrosis and haematomas. Understanding the biomechanics of the foot and lower limb will help the clinician interpret and predict these problems. Assessment of the posture and biomechanics of the musculoskeletal system is just one part of a more comprehensive assessment of the patient with haemophilia. However, it cannot be ignored as the population with haemo-philia become more active and patients, who despite prophylaxis, continue to experience bleeding episodes.

References

1 Duthie RB. Acute haemarthrosis. In: Duthie RB, Rizza CR, Giangrande PLF, Dodd CAF, eds. *The Management of Musculoskeletal Problems in the Haemophilias.* Oxford: Oxford University Press, 1994: 82–103.

2 Lehmkuhl LD, Smith LK. *Brunnstrom's Clinical Kinesiology,* 4th edn. Philadelphia: FA Davis Company, 1983.

3 White SG, Sahrmann SA. A movement system balance approach to management of musculoskeletal pain. In: Grant R, ed. *Physical Therapy of the Cervical and Thoracic Spine.* New York: Churchill Livingstone, 1994: 339–56.

4 Petty NS, Moore AP. *Neuromusculoskeletal Examination and Assessment: A Handbook for Therapists.* Edinburgh: Churchill Livingstone, 1998.

5 Donatelli R. Normal biomechanics of the foot and ankle. *J Orthop Sports Phys Ther* 1985; 7(3): 91–5.

6 Buzzard BM. Haemophilia sports injuries and physiotherapy. In: Panicucci F ed. *Let's Meet at Il Ciocco and Discuss Sport with Haemophilia.* Pisa, Italy 1992: 54–60.

7 Mannucci PM, Giangrande PLF. Management of the haemostatic defect in haemophilia. In: Duthie RB, Rizza CR, Giangrande PLF, Dodd CAF, eds. *The Management of Musculoskeletal Problems in the Haemophilias.* Oxford: Oxford University Press, 1994: 26–45.

8 Evans P. *The Knee Joint: A Clinical Guide.* Edinburgh: Churchill Livingstone, 1986.

9 Tiberio D. Pathomechanics of structural foot deformities. *Phys Ther* 1988; 68: 1840–9.

10 Subotnick SI. Biomechanics of the subtalar and midtalar joints. *J Am Podiatr Med Assoc* 1975; 65: 756–64.

11 Trickey EL. Ligamentous injuries around the knee. *BMJ* 1976; 2: 1492–4.

12 Clement DB, Taunton JE, Smart GW. Achilles tendonitis and peri tendonitis: etiology and treatment. *Am J Sports Med* 1984; 12: 179–84.

13 Ribbans WJ, Rees JL. Management of equinus contractures of the ankle in haemophilia. *Haemophilia* 1999; 5(Suppl. 1): 46–52.

14 Duthie RB, Dodd CAF. Chronic haemophilic arthropathy. In: Duthie RB, Rizza CR, Giangrande PLF, Dodd CAF, eds. *The Management of Musculoskeletal Problems in the Haemophilias.* Oxford: Oxford University Press, 1994: 159–90.

15 Heijnen L, De Kleijn P. Physiotherapy for the treatment of articular contractures in haemophilia. *Haemophilia* 1999; 5(Suppl. 1): 16–19.

16 Rodriquez-Mechan EC. Common orthopaedic problems in haemophilia. *Haemophilia* 1999; 5(Suppl. 1): 53–60.

17 Buzzard BM. Physiotherapy for the prevention of articular contraction in haemophilia. *Haemophilia* 1999; 5(Suppl. 1): 10–5.

8 Use of a Theoretical Framework for Health Status in Haemophilia Care and Research

Piet de Kleijn and Nico L.U. van Meeteren

Introduction

The life of haemophilia patients in countries where clotting factor is available, as it is in the Netherlands, has changed considerably both in quantity (duration) and in quality (health-related quality of life) [1]. In the last decade, development in haemophilia research was mainly focused on pathology, i.e. discovery of clotting factors, producing concentrates, prophylactic treatment, treatment of side-effects and, lately, recombinant products. Consequently, medical treatment has reached high standards and will probably develop towards transgenic production and gene therapy in the next decade [2].

The focus by health care practitioners on pathologies and impairments may have been a natural by-product of the exponential growth in biomedical knowledge that began in the latter half of the 20th century [3]. The 'evaluation of the non-bleeding joint' as advised in the early 1980s by the World Federation of Haemophilia (WFH), originates from that period [4]. Impairments, like muscle strength and range of motion, reflect the function of organs and organ systems. They do not necessarily reflect a person's perception of his/her capacity to live a successful life. It is our conviction that physical therapists, as many other professionals, should not deal just with pathologies and impairments, but all the more so with the disabling consequences of diseases, for instance haemophilia. Our professional colleagues committed to assisting patients towards being active participants in their own environment [3].

In this respect the understanding of the aetiology of the complex process of disablement is of major importance to haemophilia care, since only then can rehabilitation interventions be targeted properly and their effects estimated more exactly. Understanding of the disablement process can be obtained by systematic investigation, preferably guided by a sound theoretical framework [5]. In this chapter two frameworks, both dealing with the process of disablement, are introduced in a historical perspective. The overall goal of this chapter is to advocate that a theoretical framework on disablement should guide the next generation of descriptive and outcome intervention studies in haemophilia patients. Emphasis is on physical disablement because of its central role in physical therapy research and practice.

Two frameworks

To understand the complex process of disablement, one continuously has to bear in mind that theoretical frameworks simplify reality, and that the process of disablement certainly is not a linear process leading in one direction. The theoretical frameworks presented here merely represent the skeleton of the process, the 'main pathway', in which straight arrows often represent highly complex relationships. Several other frameworks and schemes have been developed, for instance for rehabilitation purposes [6], but this chapter is restricted to the World Health Organization and Nagi schemes, as these are the most commonly used [7].

WHO: International Classification of Impairments, Disabilities and Handicaps

Since 1979 the World Health Organization's (WHO) International Classification of Impairments, Disabilities and Handicaps (ICIDH) has served as a prominent framework to gain insight into the process of disablement [8]. The disablement process was used as a global term, reflecting all the array of consequences of disease, focusing on three key domains: (i) impairment; (ii) disability; and (iii) handicap. However, this framework did not serve the purposes regarding outcome assessment, certainly not when the WHO defined 'health' as a state of complete physical, mental and social well-being, and not merely the absence of disease and infirmity [9]. Gradually it became clear that the ICIDH was incomplete and that its structure needed considerable refinement. The first update, the ICIDH2, will probably be released in the year 2000 [8].

Nagi

During the 1960s the sociologist Nagi introduced his framework [10], which was recently modified by Verbrugge and Jette [7,11,12]. In this framework three domains were also defined: (i) impairment; (ii) functional limitations; and (iii) disability. The Nagi and ICIDH schemes differed when describing consequences of disease at the level of the individual, both in name and content. Jette and Verbrugge stated that 'disablement' refers to the impacts that chronic and acute conditions have on the functioning of specific body systems and on people's abilities to act in necessary, usual, expected and personally desired ways in their society. As a gap between person (capability) and environment (activity's demand), disability can be alleviated at either side, by increasing capability or by reducing demand. Unfortunately, many health care workers instinctively aim at interventions that will improve people's capabilities. To a certain extent this strategy could be the starting point, but only in perspective of an overview to both sides. In real life, efforts to reduce environmental demands are a common feature in this process.

From ICD to ICIDH2 (beta–draft)

In 1993 the International Classification of Diseases (ICD) provided a relevant means for studying health, since it was sufficient to record the occurrence of disease in either recovery or death. Nowadays conditions like diabetes and haemophilia can be controlled, even though the underlying causes cannot be eliminated. In the late 1960s the administration of disability started with assessment of functions such as activities of daily living (ADL) and instrumental activities of daily living (IADL), initially concerned with the care of the elderly. It was in the early 1970s that the WHO was interested in developing a scheme to manage consequences of disease. The principle of such a classification of long-term non-fatal consequences of disease would require a structure based on two axes at least: the individual and the interaction of the individual and environment, either physical or social. The first ICIDH was accepted as a supplement to the ICD in 1976 and eventually published in 1980. The classification was mainly built on three domains: impairment (1009 items), disability (338 items) and handicap (72 items) and is by now well established and translated into many languages [8].

During a long revision process, in April 1999 the WHO discussed the ICIDH2-beta-draft, their latest concept. In its introduction the WHO clearly states that the ICIDH represents a three-dimensional description of an individual's functional health state: (i) body (function and shape); (ii) activity; and (iii) participation (see Fig. 8.1b). Compared to the former version the difference is that the three dimensions are formulated in positive

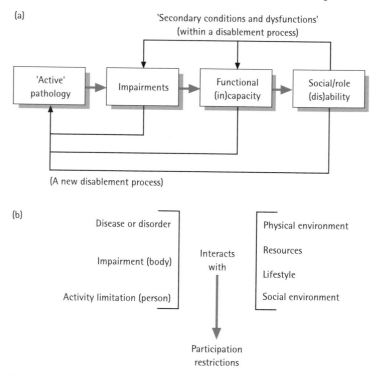

Figure 8.1 Frameworks showing the consequences of diseases, disorders or injuries. (a) Modified from Verbrugge & Jette [11] and Jette (Disablement outcomes in geriatric rehabilitation *Med Care* 35: 28–35). (b) Modified from WHO International Classification of impairments, activity and participation, Beta-1 draft for field trials.

or neutral wordings. The content of the dimensions, however, remains largely intact. For the dimension of the body, two classifications have been developed, one for functions of body systems and one for the shape of the body (and body parts). Shape does not only represent form, but also state. Shape of body parts represents, for instance, their position, presence, form and continuity. Impairments are defined as problems in body functions or shape. The dimension of activities covers the whole range of distinct activities that can be performed by an individual. Thus, a limitation in activities (formerly indicated in the ICIDH as disabilities) reflects the difficulties an individual has in performing an activity. Qualifiers serve to indicate the degree of difficulties, and the amount of assistance needed to perform the activity. A restriction in participation (formerly indicated in the ICIDH as handicap) exists when an individual has problems in one of the life domains or interacting factors [13].

Nagi and modifications (Jette, Verbrugge and Jette)

The original scheme was introduced by Nagi in the 1960s [10]. As a sociologist he was interested in non-physical consequences of pathologies. One of the most widely known extensions of his basic formulation can be found in *Disability in America: Toward a National Agenda for Prevention*, in which 'Quality of Life' was introduced as the final outcome of the process of disablement [14]. Pope and Tarlov [14] defined 'Quality of Life' as generally corresponding to total well-being, encompassing both physical and psychosocial determinants, while disability was merely seen as a precursor for outcomes such as global well-being, life satisfaction, institutionalization or even death. In 1994 Jette published a modification of the original framework of Nagi, known as 'The Disablement Process'. Jette attempted to make it more useful for physiotherapists and other health care professionals [7].

Verbrugge and Jette tried to make this more explicit (Fig. 8.1a) by recognizing 'secondary conditions and dysfunctions' and even 'a new disablement process' [11]. The term 'secondary conditions' is used by the Institute of Medicine to cover all feedback effects, whether they involve pathology, impairment, functional limitation or disability [14]. Verbrugge and Jette [11] distinguished feedback effects that occur within a particular disablement process from those that launch new pathology.

Verbrugge and Jette [11] introduced intra-individual and extra-individual factors, and risk factors as influencing factors of the process of disability. Jette states: 'An important question for disability research is to identify the extent to which identified disabilities in selected populations are the result of social and physical environment in contrast to factors within the individual' [7]. Intra-individual factors could be lifestyle and behaviour changes, coping or activity accommodations (changes in kinds of activities, but also in frequency or length of time doing them). Extra-individual factors consist for instance of co-interventions or physical and social environment (like employment discrimination, structural modifications at home, health insurance, access to medical care, etc.). Disablement risk factors usually exist prior to the onset of active pathology and may exist in behaviours, attributes, or environmental influences that elevate the chances of developing impairments, functional limitations, or disability [11]. Changes have been made towards positive terms, as also seen in the ICIDH (see Fig. 8.1a) [12].

Epidemiology (aetiology of the process of disablement)

(From here onwards the authors will use terms from the ICIDH2 proposals.)

Cure and prevention of disability in general has emerged as a major societal concern. The development of effective disability intervention strategies must be preceded by careful unravelling of the process of disablement, using well defined epidemiology and outcome measures [12]. To unravel this process several descriptive studies, using either the ICIDH or the Nagi framework have been carried out, as in juvenile chronic arthritis, osteogenesis imperfecta, multitrauma patients and elderly people suffering from osteoarthritis. By means of these studies insight was gained into the dynamic characteristics, natural course, basic mechanisms and complex causal relations between impairments, activities and participation of these patient populations [15,16]. For instance, Van der Net *et al.* demonstrated that in children suffering from polyarticular juvenile chronic arthritis positive inflammation parameters were present in the blood for 25% of them. Their joints, however, only showed slight impairments like pain and swelling, although their functions, as measured with the

'Juvenile Arthritis Functional Assessment Scale', were limited in a much more severe way [17]. The perception of these children, concerning activities of daily living and general health, was less pronounced. Correlation analysis between the domains of 'the disablement process' proved mutual interactions between impairments and activities, but not between active pathology and impairments, neither between activities and participation [18]. The outcome of Van der Net *et al.* correspond to those of many others: the general conclusion is that, with respect to the disability process, we deal with a highly complex, dynamic and nonlinear process. We concur with others that probably there is no one-to-one relation-ship between the disability phenomena and their optional intervention strategies.

Translation to haemophilia care and research

The 'disablement process' is complex in nature and it seems that this holds true for haemophilia patients as well. This is substantiated by a large study of Triemstra and coworkers. A questionnaire 'Haemophilia in the Netherlands', version 4 (HIN4), returned by 980 Dutch haemophilia patients out of a total of 1400 provided in-depth insight into the mutual relationships between the severity of haemophilia, impairments and perceived level of activities. The conclusion of the HIN4 was that the self perception of well-being has no linear relation with the severity of haemophilia [1]. Further research by Triemstra demonstrated that psychological factors are the strongest determinants of well being [19], which is consistent with outcomes in rheumatoid arthritis research. In general, perceptions of well being and quality of life of different patient populations is more positive than one should estimate. This may have to do with the balance patients rate between body, mind and spirit in the self and on establishing and maintaining a harmonious set of relationships within a person's social context and external environment [20].

All in all, it seems that complexity is apparent at each level and stage of the disablement process. Complexity in haemophilia is even more impressive when considering interacting factors and feedback loops. Interacting factors (see Fig. 8.1b) seem of decisive importance in haemophilia care world-wide. In these patients medical care is a highly relevant example of an extra-individual factor, since patients' fate is so much dependent on the availability of medicine (i.e. clotting factor). Demographic context, like living in developing countries is an important example of a risk factor to haemophilia patients, not only because of the lack of clotting factor, but for many other reasons, like poor transportation facilities to reach a hospital or haemophilia centre. Personal assistance (parents to perform home treatment for their child) or special equipment and devices (to perform home treatment), both examples of external supports, differ amongst patients. In view of the apparent relevance of the aforementioned interacting factors we recommend identification and vigorous assessment of these in haemophilia disablement research.

As can be seen in Fig. 8.1(a), several 'feedback loops' exist within a disablement process. Such a feedback loop is represented by a haemophilia patient, having arthropathic, painful joints, restricting his/her recreational walking (participation), eventually inducing muscle weakness (feedback to impairment), further reducing mobility and social activities (feedback to activity and participation).

Future research

From an epidemiological point of view, physical therapists need adequate tools to be able to measure relevant items in each domain and describe the natural course of a disease and its consequences. To study the natural course of diseases and disability consequences, longitudinal research is required, with relevant tools for this purpose. Longitudinal research in rheumatoid arthritis (RA) for instance identified that disabilities mainly developed during the first six years of the disease [21]. In osteoarthritis research several international institutions reached a high degree of consensus on a core set of measures (OMERACT III) in knee, hip and hand osteoarthritis clinical trials. Included in this core set were measurements of pain, physical function, patient global examination and radiological imaging [22]. Longitudinal research in haemophilia has as yet, rarely been carried out, and certainly not in the perspective of the 'disability process'. Therefore our group started a strategy in order to propel the discussion on a new WFH measurement standard [23].

In 1982 the WFH advised the 'evaluation of the non-bleeding

joint', scoring: bleeding frequency, pain, clinical and radiological parameters [4]. Besides the fact that not all of these have been proven scientifically valid within the haemophilia population, these measures focus almost exclusively on 'active' pathology (bleeding frequency) and impairments (pain, clinical score and Pettersson score), whereas the whole 'disability process' would be preferred. However, up until now no disease-specific, reliable and valid instruments have been developed and evaluated on impairments (of body), activities and participation. A few attempts have been made, for instance Iwata evaluated activities of daily living in haemophilia patients in Japan with help from a questionnaire [24]. Others evaluated existing tools like the Health Assessment Questionnaire [25], the Arthritis Impact and Measurement Scales-2, and Canadian Occupational Perform-ance Measure [26–28]. In the near future these developments will hopefully result in an up-to-date 'WFH-2 score', consisting of reliable and validated tools that properly measure relevant items in all domains of the disability process of haemophilia patients.

Conclusion

The common pathway of epidemiological approach and theore-tical constructs, whether the ICIDH2 or modified Nagi frame-work, possibly provide better insight in the 'aetiology of disablement'. This may lead towards exploration of (possible) causal relations and determinants of disablement, also in a longitudinal perspective. Besides descriptive and outcome research by means of reliable and valid instruments to measure all domains, longitudinal research in haemophilia patients is needed to unravel disability consequences of the disease haemo-philia, of which medical treatment has changed so rapidly over the last decades. Comparing different age groups is one way to do so [29,30]. The focus on older haemophilia patients suffering from severe painful elbow, knee or ankle joints has changed towards youngsters, limited in their functioning because of one arthropathic ankle [31] and towards the under-10s, who may suffer more from mental and social effects rather than physical consequences of their disease. Therefore the value of variable risk factors remains of major importance; predisposing, intra-and extra-individual risk factors may influence this dynamic process of disablement in haemophilia patients. There is a long, but necessary way to go for those of us bearing full responsibility for the haemophilia patients entrusted to our care.

References

1   Triemstra AMH, Ploeg v.d. HM, Smit C, Briet E, Rosendaal FR. *Hemofilie in Nederland 4*. Amsterdam-VU Leiden-RUL/AZL, 1999.

2   O'Mahony B. Plasma-derived and biotech products: what is the future of haemophilia therapy? *Occasional Papers World Federation of Haemophilia (WFH)*, Montreal 1999.

3   Rothstein JM, Scalzitti DA. Commentary: physiotherapy *quo vadis*. *Adv Physiotherapy* 1999; 1: 9–12.

4   Gilbert MS. Prophylaxis: musculoskeletal evaluation. *Semin Hematol* 1993; 30: 3–6.

5   Alderson P. The importance of theories in health care. *Education Debate* 1998; 317: 1007–10.

6   Post MWM. Quality of life and the ICIDH: towards an integrated conceptual model for rehabilitation outcomes research. *Clin Rehab* 1999; 13: 5–15.

7   Jette AM. Physical disablement concepts for physical therapy research and practice. *Phys Ther* 1994; 74: 380–6.

8   Thuriaux MC. The ICIDH. evolution, status, and prospects. *Disabil Rehabil* 1995; 17: 112–18.

9   WHO. *The First Ten Years of the World Health Organization*. Geneva 1958.

10 Nagi S. Some conceptual issues in disability and rehabilitation. *Sociology and Rehabilitation* 1965; 100–13.

11 Verbrugge LM, Jette AM. The disablement process. *Soc Sci Med* 1994; 38: 2–13.

12 Jette AM. Disentangling the process of disablement. *Soc Sci Med* 1999; 48: 471–2.

13 Halbertsma J. The revision of the ICIDH introduction. *Newsletter RIVM* 1999; 2: 1–2.

14 Pope A, Tarlov A. *Disability in America: Toward a National Agenda for Prevention*. Washington DC: National Academy Press, 1991.

15 Helders PJM, Engelbert RHH, Net v.d. J, Gulmans VAM. Physiotherapy *quo vadis*: towards an evidence-based, diagnosis-related, functional approach. *Adv Physiotherapy* 1999; 1: 3–7.

16 Van Meeteren NLU, Verhoef J, Net v.d. J, Helders PJM. Systematisch ordenen en begrijpen van het 'disablement process': conditio sine qua non voor verdere ontwikkeling van de fysiotherapie. (Systematic approach and understanding of the 'disablement process': conditio sine qua non for future development in physiotherapy). *Nederlands Tijdschrift Voor Fysiotherapie* 1999; 129: 54–7.

17 Van der Net J, Hoeven H, Esseveld v.d. F, Wilde EJD, Kuis W, Helders PJM. Musculoskeletal disorders in juvenile mixed connective tissue disease. *J Rheumatol* 1995; 22: 751–7.

18 Helders PJM, Net v.d. J, Engelbert RHH. Functionele diagnostiek: Een semantische of inhoudelijke discussie? (Functional diagnostics: semantic or in depth discussion?). *Tijdschrift voor oefentherapie-Mensendieck* 1998; 3: 28–35.

19 Triemstra AMH. Well being of haemophilia patients: a model for direct and indirect effects of medical parameters on the physical and psychosocial functioning. *Soc Sci Med* 1998; 47: 581–93.

20 Albrecht GL, Devlieger PJ. The disability paradox: high quality of life against all odds. *Soc Sci Med* 1999; 48: 977–88.

21 Van Jaarsveld CMH, Jacobs JWG, Schrijvers AJP, Albada-Kuipers GA, Hofman DM, Bijlsma JWJ. Effects of rheumatoid arthritis on employment and social participation during the first years of disease in the Netherlands. *Br J Rheumatol* 1998; 37: 848–53.

22 Bellamy N, Kirwan J, Boers M *et al*. Recommendations for a Core Set of Outcome Measures for Future Phase III Clinical Trials in Knee, Hip, and Hand Osteoarthritis. Consensus Development at OMERACT III. *J Rheumatol* 1997; 24: 799–802.

23 De Kleijn P, Mauser-Bunschoten EP, Roosendaal G *et al*. Regarding the 'disablement process' in hemophilia. In: Lusher JM, Kessler CM, eds. *Hemophilia and Von Willebrand's Disease in the 1990s*, 943 edn. 1999, 201–4.

24 Iwata N, Hachisuka K, Tanaka S, Naka Y, Ogata H. Measuring activities of daily living among haemophiliacs. *Dis Rehab* 1996; 18: 217–23.

25 Cornwell EJ, Scott GL, Atkins RM. *Changes in Musculoskeletal Disability in Haemophilia following the use of a Dedicated Haemophilic Physiotherapist*. 21st International Congress of the World Federation of Haemophilia, Mexico City, April 24–29, 1994. (Abstract.)

26 Van Meeteren NLU, De Joode E, De Kleijn P, Van den Berg HM, Helders PJM. Evaluation of activities and participation in hemophilia patients: validity of the Dutch AIMS2. 1999. (Submitted.)

27 Van Meeteren NLU, Effing T, Strato I, Sleegers EJA, Helders PJM. Evaluation and implementation of the Canadian Occupational Performance Measure (COPM) in rehabilitation. *Dis Rehab* (in press).

28 Van Meeteren NLU, Strato I, Veldhoven NHMJV, Kleijn P, van den Berg HM, Helders PJM. Usefulness of the D-AIMS2 for measurement of health status in Dutch hemophilia patients. *Haemophilia*, (submitted).

29 Fischer K, van den Berg HM, Mauser Bunschoten EP, Roosendaal G. 1999 Changing treatment strategies for severe hemophilia A; on clinical outcome and costs. A pilot study. Poster ASH 1997.

30 Lofqvist T, Nilsson IM, Petersson C. Orthopaedic surgery in hemophilia. 20 years' experience in Sweden. *Clin Orthop* 1996; 332: 232–41.

31 Buzzard BM, Heim M. A study to evaluate the effectiveness of 'Air-Stirrup' splints as a means of reducing the frequency of ankle haemarthroses in children with haemophilia A and B. *Haemophilia* 1995; 1: 131–6.

9   Disability and Outcome Measures in Patients with Haemophilia

Jane Cornwell

Introduction

There is much pressure on health workers to improve clinical effectiveness and efficiency and set standards for good practice. World-wide economic constraints on health care systems have stressed the need to monitor the outcomes of care and output of the health system. The information offered by outcomes research can provide this and ensuring this information is correct can be crucial to those with haemophilia as well as the health service as a whole.

Due to the increased need for outcome measures, a wide range of measures have been generated which are designed to estimate the need for health care and the outcomes of such health care. The majority have been developed in the USA where the pressure to develop effectiveness and efficiency has been much emphasized. There are vast quantities of published material and a large number of available measures in the area of measuring physical disability and handicap. A single outcome measurement tool does not exist as it would be impossible to have one measurement to assess disability, pain and impact of disability on one's life. It would also be incorrect to develop a set of questions suited to all individuals and diseases, as a particular instrument would have to note so many compromises that it would not be suitable for any particular disease as there would be too many variants. Therefore in order to ensure the outcome measurements used are relevant and sensitive to the group of people it is administered to, it is advisable to choose the most appropriate outcome measurement tool available. This is a daunting task due to the amount of material available [1]. This article outlines the benefits and limitations of two extensively used outcome measurement tools namely the Health Assessment Questionnaire (HAQ) [2] and the Arthritis Impact Measurement Scales (AIMS) [3] which have both been used in clinical practice in patients with haemophilia.

Choosing the relevant measurement tool

A systematic review of previously developed measurement tools has identified that there is no available validated disability outcome questionnaire/measurement tool specifically for patients with haemophilia. The World Federation of Haemophilia Scoring System exists to assess pain (grade 0–3), haemorrhage incidence in any one year (grade 0–3) and instability (grade 0–2). Whilst these are useful measurements, they do not provide an outcome measurement on how a patient with haemophilia copes with his or her disability both physically and emotionally and cannot necessarily give an accurate indication of ability of performance and the patient's subjective feelings and their reduction in activities associated with daily living [4]. It would seem more appropriate that in order to review and monitor haemophilia health status, disease progression, administration of factor replacement therapy, medical and surgical intervention, physiotherapy and pain control, to name a few modalities, that not only should the World Federation of Haemophilia (WFH) scoring system be used but also that outcome measurements for disability and the effects of disability should be evaluated. These outcome measurements if standardized could be administered and used by those in contact with patients with haemophilia to aid in the assessment of the effectiveness of treatment given and to review disease progression and the needs of the patient with haemophilia.

As suggested, developing an instrument that accurately measures patient outcome is difficult. Many considerations need to be taken into account before the most appropriate measurement tool can be used. In the field of measurements specific to health care, basic physical function has the character of minimum standards; they define basic functions (e.g. walking, dressing, working) which all adult human beings should be able to perform for themselves; these definitions of need can be very limited. By focusing on what is easily measurable they can ignore what people regard as real or legitimate needs. There are differences between cultures and even between groups within the same culture, which can result in a measure being appropriate or not which needs to be considered. When measuring function then activities of daily living (ADL) are dealt with, with the purpose of describing the impact of chronic disease/illness on the lives of the patients and the impact of the chronic disease in terms of the restrictions it places on the ability of the individuals to lead normal lives [5].

When faced with choosing the most specific functional outcome for patients with haemophilia it seems most appropriate to look at disease specific measures. Specialists in the treatment of arthritic diseases have devoted considerable efforts to the problems of defining and measuring outcomes of treatment. The Fries Stanford Health Assessment Questionnaire (HAQ) [2] and the Meenans arthritic impact measurement scales (AIMS) [3] have been developed to meet a need for outcome measures in the field of arthritic disease. They have similar levels of reliability and validity. These two disability outcome measurement tools are discussed following some necessary definitions.

Definitions

The WHO has described alterations in function as three progressive stages termed impairment, disability and handicap.

1 *Impairment* refers to the reduction in physical or mental capacities which may not be visible or may not be detrimental for the individual. If impairment is not corrected a disability may result.

2 *Disability* refers to a restriction in a person's ability to perform a function in a manner considered normal for a human being (e.g. to walk). Disability may or may not limit the individual's ability to fulfil a normal social role, depending on its severity and on what the person wishes to do.

3 *Handicap* refers to social disadvantage (e.g. loss of earnings) that may arise from disability.

The Health Assessment Questionnaire aims to assess the impact of disability, but also the direct and indirect economic effects of the illness/disease, i.e. part of handicap [5].

Validity and reliability

The analogy used to describe the validity and reliability of a measurement has been described as someone learning archery who must first learn to hit the centre of the target and then learn to do this consistently [5,6]. The reliability (or consistency) would be represented by the aim of the shooting, on average how close successive shots fall to each other, whenever they land on the target. Validity would be represented by the aim of the shooting, on average how close the shots are at the centre of the target. Reliable and valid would be a close group of shots at the centre of the target. In short validity is concerned with whether the indicator (e.g. disability index) does measure what it claims to and reliability (or consistency) is judged when the measure consistently produces the same results, especially when administered by different observers and at different times. A disability measurement tool should also be sensitive, i.e. detect changes in the patient's condition. This explanation of validity and reliability has been much simplified and a great deal more can be read on this subject [4,5].

Most measures of functional disability are self report methods, this method can also obtain the subjective assessment of experiences (e.g. feelings about level of health and well being) [4]. They are often quick to administer and involve little interpretation by the investigator. To date it has proved useful to administer both the HAQ and the AIMS to patients with haemophilia. The HAQ measures specific measures of physical function and activity limitations and this includes for example hand dexterity which may not be very sensitive to the patient with haemophilia. The AIMS provides information on the impact of the disease. The correlation of 0.91 between the HAQ and AIMS is remarkably high [7]. It has been suggested that application of more than one measurement is advisable as it can reinforce conclusions of a study and can increase our understanding of the comparability of the measurements [5].

The Health Assessment Questionnaire

The Health Assessment Questionnaire (HAQ) measures difficulty in performing activities of daily living. Originally used in adult patients with arthritis, it has since been used extensively in the research setting to evaluate care. The disability section of the HAQ comprises of 20 questions on daily functioning during the past week. These cover eight areas: dressing and grooming, arising, eating, walking, hygiene, reach, grip and outdoor activities. The scale may be self administered, or given in an interview or on the telephone. It can be completed in 5–8 min and scored in 1 min. Each response is scored on a four point scale of ability, which ranges from 'without any difficulty' to 'unable to do', a check list records any aids used or assistance received. The HAQ has been used extensively and there is considerable evidence of validity and reliability. It is available in a shortened form known as the 'modified HAQ' [8] and there is an 'AIDS-HAQ'. The HAQ has also been adapted for use in many countries including Britain [9], when it was demonstrated that some of the questions phased in a North American style confused some British patients and hindered completion and understanding of the questionnaire. Once modified it indicated it was more sensitive to change. This was the version used in the study with haemophilia [10] patients in the UK. The HAQs design offers a scale which consists of a broad scope but brief enough for easy and quick completion. The criticisms focus on the simplicity of the scoring system which may be at the cost of precision.

The Arthritis Impact Measurement Scales

This combines measurements of physical functioning with social and emotional aspects of health. This type of health measurement score is known as 'general health status measures', 'measures of health related to quality of life' or 'quality of life measures'. The Arthritis Impact Measurement Scales (AIMS) covers physical, social and emotional well being and was originally designed as an indicator of outcome of care for patients with arthritis. It consists of 45 items grouped into nine scales that assess mobility, physical activity, dexterity, household activity, social activity, activities of daily living, pain and depression. The items included were analysed by the Guttman Scaling (scalogram analysis) and demonstrated interval consistency correlation [3] and for each scale the items are listed in Guttman order. Most questions refer to problems during the past month. In scoring the AIMS each item is scored separately, ignoring the Guttman characteristics, higher scores indicate greater limitation. Details of scoring are provided in a user's guide available from the Boston Arthritis Centre [11]. The AIMS has been translated into various languages and the abbreviated version includes 18 items divided into 9 scales, which takes 6–8 min to complete. AIMS2 is also now used extensively and has its own users guide [12]. The AIMS has also been used with children (average age 9.3 years) with mixed success. The AIMS has extensively demonstrated its validity and reliability. It can be completed on interview or self administered and takes approximately 15 min. It has been noted that the AIMS deserves serious consideration as an outcome indicator for patients with arthritic disease [5].

Use of HAQ and AIMS

There are many references on the use of the HAQ and the AIMS when used together or separately. They were shown to be sensitive to change in physical function when administered prior to joint replacement surgery [13]. They have also been used to evaluate outcome in patients who have undergone total knee replacement [14]. The AIMS was used in a study to compare the effects of physical therapy prior to total knee replacement compared to no physical therapy [15]. It also demonstrated sensitivity to improvements in OA and RA produced by non-steroidal anti-inflammatory drugs [16]. The use of the HAQ and AIMS2 indicated the benefits of hydrotherapy with patients with arthritic disease [17,18]. The HAQ was used in a study to measure outcomes of self help education for patients with arthritis [19]. It was also used to compare patients with knee osteoarthritis (OA) who had back pain with those who did not have back pain [20]. The two questionnaires were used in a study with patients with rheumatic disease and demonstrated that they provided valid means of helping to identify their needs appropriately [21].

Application in haemophilia

In the study of the use of a Flowtron intermittent pressure garment in the treatment of fixed flexion deformities in patients with haemophilia [22], the HAQ was administered to the patients to self complete pre and post application of the Flowtron pressure garment. The HAQ score did indicate some significant change but it was noted that there were areas of the HAQ that were insensitive to patients with haemophilia, e.g. the dexterity and grip components, and that it would have been more appropriate (i.e. sensitive) to include activities that used elbow movement (pronation/supination, flexion/extension). Such subjective data is useful information for a possible future disability index for patients with haemophilia.

Physiotherapy application in haemophilia

The HAQ and the AIMS were both used in a more recent study [10] when a physiotherapist was employed solely for the purpose of treating patients with haemophilia for their musculoskeletal problems. The funding was provided initially by a grant from the British Haemophilia Society. There had been no regular dedicated physiotherapy for these patients in the past. The patients were seen on a regular basis by the physiotherapist and treated as clinically indicated. Assessment measurements included joint range of movement (ROM) and fixed flexion deformity (FFD) and the administration of the HAQ and AIMS at regular intervals. These two were chosen after extensive reading and research. The results included an overall significant reduction in FFD in elbows and knees, accompanied by overall significant increase in joint ROM; these results relapsed with the interruption of physiotherapy for eight weeks and improved again with the re-introduction of physiotherapy. Both the HAQ and the AIMS scores (including each component of the AIMS) demonstrated a statistically significant improvement with physiotherapy treatment. These outcome results were an essential component of ensuring that this physiotherapy position became permanent and was funded by the purchasers of health care for the future benefit of care for patients with haemophilia. This demonstrates the use of disability outcome measurements in helping to provide improved haemophilia care.

Conclusion

The need and emphasis on controlling health care costs and hence the stimulus for research into effectiveness and efficiency of health services is a world-wide issue. The care of the patient with haemophilia is a part of this and in order to provide the most appropriate care available to these patients outcome measurements are an essential component of management. To date no specific disability, disease impact measurement tool is available for patients with haemophilia. Although it would seem difficult to provide such a measurement tool it needs to be seriously considered when assessing the need for care in patients with haemophilia. Therefore testing existing instruments and possibly refining them is necessary. Decisions affecting the welfare of patients, including those with haemophilia, and expenditure of public funds are based on the results of health measurements, and pressures to monitor outcomes of treatment are essential. This chapter has highlighted the need for the use of a physical disability measure and the impact of disability outcome measurement tools for patients with haemophilia, in order to monitor their disease and evaluate the treatment aimed at improving their care. It suggests two measures that have been used to date on such patients. Disability and its impact outcome measurements provide many uses. They can help identify best practice and development of practice guidelines and can aid in clinical decision making. They can provide information for resource allocation and other policy decisions and if used on a national or international basis could help to provide some scientific evidence to assist in the care of patients with haemophilia in the future [23].

References

1 Wilkin D, Hallam L, Doggett M-A. *Measures of Need and Outcome for Primary Healthcare*. Oxford: Medical Publications, 1992.
2 Fries JF, Spitz P, Kraines RG *et al*. Measurement of patient outcome in arthritis. *Arthritis Rheum* 1980; 23: 137–45.
3 Meenan RF. The AIMS approach to health status measurement: conceptual background and measurement properties. *J Rheumatol* 1982; 9: 785–8.
4 Bowling A. *Measuring Health*. Open University Press, 1991.
5 McDowell I, Newell C. *Measuring Health*, 2nd edn. Oxford: Oxford University Press , 1996.
6 Ahlborn A. Nurells Introduction to Modern Epidemiology Chestnut Hill, Montana, 1984.
7 Brown JH, Kazis LE, Spitz PW *et al*. The dimensions of health outcomes: a cross validated examination of health status measurement. *AmJ Public Health* 1984; 74: 159–61.

8   Pincus T, Callahan LF, Brooks RH *et al*. Self report questionnaire scores in rheumatoid arthritis compared with traditional, physical, radiographic and laboratory measures. *Ann Intern Med* 1989; 110: 259–66.

9   Kirwan JR, Reeback JS. Standford Health Assessment Questionnaire modified to assess disability in British patients with rheumatoid arthritis. *Br J Rheum* 1986; 25: 206–9.

10 Cornwell J, Scott G, Atkins RA. The use of a dedicated physiotherapist in the treatment of patients with haemophilia. *Haemophilia* (submitted).

11 Boston University Multipurpose Arthritis Centre. *AIMS Users Guide*. Boston: Boston University.

12 Meenon RF, Mason JH, Anderson JJ. AIMS 2: the content and properties of a revised and expected arthritis impact measurement scales. Health status questionnaire. *Arthritis Rheum* 1992; 35: 1–10.

13 Goeppinger J, Thomas Doyle MA, Charlton SL, Loria K. A nursing perspective on assessment of function in person with arthritis. *Res Nursing Health* 1988; 11: 321–31.

14 Lang MH, Fossel AH, Larson MG. Comparisons of five health status instruments for orthopaedic evaluation. *Med Care* 1990; 28: 632–42.

15 Lima D, Colwell CW, Morris BA, Harwick ME. The effect of pre-operative exercise on total knee replacement outcomes. *Clin Orthop* 1996; 362: 174–82.

16 Andeson J, Hill E, Meenan RF *et al*. Sensitivity of a health status measure to short term clinical changes in arthritis. *Arthritis Rheum* 1989; 32(7): 844–50.

17 Hall J, Skevington SM, Maddison PJ, Chapman K. A randomised and controlled trial of hydrotherapy in rheumatoid arthritis. *Arthritis Care Research* 1996; 9: 206–15.

18 Sanford-Smith S, Mackay-Lyons M, Nunes-Clement S. Therapeutic benefit of aquaerobics for individuals with rheumatoid arthritis. *Physiother Can* 1998; 50: 40–6.

19 Lorig K, Lubeck D, Kraines RG *et al*. Outcomes of self help education for patients with arthritis. *Arthritis Rheum* 1985; 28: 680–5.

20 Wolfe F, Hawley DJ, Peloso PM, Wilson K. Back pain in osteoarthritis of the knee. *Arthritis Care Res* 1996; 9: 376–83.

21 Hill J. Health status in rheumatic disease. *Nurs Stand* 1991; 6: 25–7.

22 Yates P, Cornwell J, Atkins RM *et al*. Treatment of haemophiliac flexion deformity using the flowtron intermittent compression system. *Br J Haematol* 1992; 82: 384–7.

23 Delamothe T, ed. Outcomes into Clinical Practice. BMJ Publishing Group.

10 Orthopaedic Surgery in Haemophilia

E. Carlos Rodriguez-Merchan

Introduction

Over 90% of bleeding episodes in people with haemophilia occur within the musculoskeletal system and of these, 80% occur within the joints. The management of orthopaedic problems in patients with haemophilia requires a haematologist, whose function is to control haemostasis, an orthopaedic surgeon, a physical therapist, an orthotist and an occupational therapist, all of whom concentrate on the preservation and restoration of function of the musculoskeletal system. The most important component of management in patients with haemophilia is the avoidance of recurrent haemarthroses by means of haematological prophylaxis. Continuous prophylactic clotting factor replacement from the ages of 2–18 years prevents the development of haemophilic arthropathy if the concentration of the patient's deficient factor is prevented from falling below 1% of normal.

Unfortunately this is not currently possible in the majority of countries around the world. When only on-demand haematological treatment is available, the frequent occurrence of intra-articular bleeding episodes can lead to chronic synovitis and haemophilic arthropathy. Once arthropathy develops the functional prognosis is poor. This chapter is an overview of the diagnosis and surgical treatment of the most important problems for the patient with haemophilia: haemarthroses, synovitis, articular contractures, angular deformities and haemophilic arthropathy. The main non-articular problems of haemophilia will also be reviewed: muscular haematomas and pseudotumours. This chapter is based on experience of the orthopaedic treatment of haemophilia patients over the last 25 years.

Bleeds within the joints and synovitis

With the early provision of the missing coagulation factor, hae-morrhages can be controlled and conservative management can usually terminate the episode without any long-term complica-tions. Should the haemorrhage persist or a re-bleed occur, the synovium begins to hypertrophy and a vicious circle of chronic synovitis develops, leading to joint destruction and the classical haemophilic arthropathy. If continuous prophylaxis is not fea-sible due to expense or lack of venous access, then a major hae-marthrosis must be aggressively treated as follows: transfusion at 50%, joint aspiration, short-term immobilization for 3–5 days and transfusion every 48 hours until the joint is fully rehabili-tated. The latter requires 20–30 days of transfusion. The author believes in the efficacy of early joint aspiration of haemophilic haemarthroses. Such a technique must be done under haema-tological control and aseptic conditions. The procedure must be repeated many times in the patient's life, starting at a very young age and it carries some difficulties from the practical point of view; therefore psychological and family support are para-mount. It is important that the child trusts the orthopaedic sur-geon carrying out the procedure and it should be done with some form of local anaesthesia in order to minimize pain [1]. Follow-ing the procedure, immobilization is recommended for 3–5 days by means of a compressive bandage. Later on, the patient should start a supervised period of physiotherapy as rehabilitation is of paramount importance to halt the development of a synovitis.

Synovitis causes hypertrophy of the epiphyseal plates. Bone hypertrophy may lead to leg length discrepancies, angular deformities and alterations of contour in the developing skele-ton. If the synovitis is not controlled, cartilage damage will follow. As the joint cartilage progressively degrades, deteriora-tion in joint function occurs. Symptoms of chronic arthropathy typically develop by the second or third decade [2]. Ultra-sonography and/or magnetic resonance imaging are required in order to confirm the diagnosis of synovitis. There are a number of procedures designed for synovial destruction such as: syno-viorthesis (medical synovectomy) with some chemical or radio-active substances, and surgical synovectomy by open or arthroscopic technique [3]. There is still controversy on which type of synovectomy is better.

Synoviorthesis is a common therapeutic procedure for chronic haemophilic synovitis. However, controversy exists regarding the optimal age and stage of the disease for use of such drugs. In the author's opinion, synoviorthesis under local anaesthesia with Yttrium-90 should be the first choice, and could be repeated every 3 months. If after three synoviorthesis treatments, the state of synovitis has not improved sufficiently then arthroscopic synovectomy is indicated. It is recommended that the procedure should be performed in young children and in joints having 0–2 points on the radiographic score of Pettersson and Gilbert [4]. When the radiographic score is >2 points, synoviorthesis is not appropriate; instead, arthroscopic synovectomy is indicated. Open synovectomy is also effective, but at the expense of significant loss of movement.

Articular contractures and angular deformities

Joint flexion contractures in haemophilia are common and difficult problems to solve when they become fixed. Once they occur it is essential to solve them as soon as possible. In the author's opinion, the surgeon should correct the flexion contracture to prevent the degenerative changes that articular malalignment will produce in the future. At the knee this can be achieved by means of soft tissue procedures such as hamstring tenotomy and post-erior capsulotomy. At the ankle joint, an Achilles tendon lengthening and posterior capsulotomy has also been described as a useful procedure. In more severe contractures, osteotomies around the knee and ankle are indicated. Progressive extension of the joints by means of circular external fixators has been recently used with encouraging results. Some types of orthoses have been designed for progressive extension, and above all to maintain an adequate degree of extension once it has been regained. As already stated, an uncontrolled synovitis will lead to valgus or varus deviation caused by asymmetrical growth of the epiphyses. For this, in infants, adolescents and young adults, realignment osteotomies may be indicated to prevent development of severe arthropathy. Encouraging results have been reported at the knee and the ankle. Proximal tibial valgus osteotomy is an effective and reliable treatment method for painful genu varum of the haemophilic knee.

Haemophilic arthropathy

The most characteristic radiographic findings of haemophilic arthropathy are subchondral cysts, osteoporosis, enlarged epiphyses, irregular subchondral surface, narrowing of the joint space, erosions of the joint margin, gross incongruence of the articulating bone ends and joint deformity (angulation and/or displacement between articulating bones). In the final stages fibrous or osseous ankylosis will take place. The most important difference between haemophilic arthropathy and idiopathic osteoarthritis is the lack of correlation between pain and the radiographic signs. Many people with haemophilia will present with severe joint destruction over many years with little or no pain.

The surgical treatment of haemophilic arthropathy is always symptomatic, and will depend on the degree of pain and functional impairment. In its final stages in adult patients a total joint arthroplasty may be indicated, especially at the shoulder, elbow, hip and knee. In young adults and adolescents there are some surgical techniques that can be performed other than total joint replacement: resection of the radial head and partial synovectomy to improve elbow pronation–supination; knee joint debridement to delay a total knee replacement; osteotomies around the knee or ankle for varus or valgus malalignments; and currettage and bone filling, with cancellous bone and fibrin seal of some large subchondral cysts. At the ankle some patients develop a large anterior osteophyte; surgical excision of this can give relief of symptoms [5].

Arthrodesis of the shoulder has proved to be a good and reliable procedure. In patients with haemophilia, however, where elbow joint destruction and limitation of movement are so common, this procedure must be more critically reviewed. Total shoulder arthroplasty remains controversial. At the elbow joint, excision of the radial head and partial open synovectomy is a well-documented procedure. The use of total elbow joint replacement is not yet an accepted form of therapy and hence two options remain; the use of an orthotic brace or arthrodesis. End-stage haemophilic arthropathy necessitating arthroplasty is infrequent in the hip (Fig. 10.1). Although results are inferior to those obtained in arthrosis, total hip replacement should be considered in haemophilia patients [6]. Kelley *et al.* [7] reported a

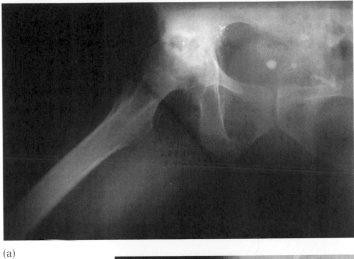

(a)

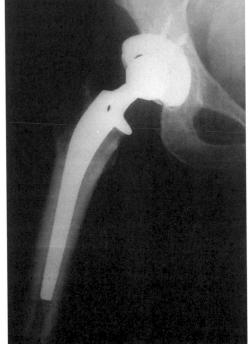

(b)

Figure 10.1 (a) Radiographs of a 42-year-old man with severe haemophilic arthropathy and (b) at eight years after a hybrid total hip arthroplasty.

high rate of loosening of the cemented hip prostheses in patients with haemophilia. There was also a high overall rate of mortality and a high rate of late deep infection in patients who were seropositive for the human immunodeficiency virus (HIV).

Smith *et al.* [8] proposed that angular deformities in the lower limbs placed a varus or valgus strain on the knee joint and that this malalignment was the trigger for the haemarthroses. Based upon this theory, osteotomies were carried out on the long bones. Total knee replacements in relatively young patients hold intrinsic dangers of prosthetic loosening and late joint infections in immunologically compromised people. Debridement should be considered in the young haemophilia patient to delay total knee arthroplasty. The operation may give the patient years of life without pain [9]. Supramalleolar varus osteotomy has been reported for haemophilic arthropathy and secondary valgus deformity. The procedure is an attractive alternative to the more commonly used surgical option of arthrodesis [10].

Intramuscular bleeds and pseudotumours

In the majority of cases, bleeds within the muscles are caused by trauma. They are very often associated with direct trauma and the pathology becomes quite evident due to the swelling, pain, local warmth and frequently a bruise in the overlying skin. The vast majority of these intramuscular bleeds resolve spontaneously, leaving no functional loss. It is, however, necessary to examine the patient carefully to ensure that there is no danger to vascular elements or neural compromise [11]. With appropriate haematological treatment, the haematomas will be reabsorbed but there is a tendency for recurrence. Thus, treatment should be maintained for several weeks until the bleed has totally resolved. Generally speaking, any haematoma should be monitored and treated long term with factor coverage.

It is paramount to ensure that complete reabsorption has occurred to avoid the risk of the development of a pseudotumour. Another risk is the haematogenous spontaneous infection of the haematoma. In people with haemophilia, a positive HIV status is strongly related to septic arthritis and there is also a high risk of developing full-blown AIDS. Septic arthritis provides a clinical marker for immunodepression in patients with haemophilia. It is important to remember that a painful and swollen joint, mimicking haemarthrosis, could be due to septic arthritis especially when factor replacement fails to relieve the symptoms and there is pyrexia. This requires prompt diagnosis and antibiotic therapy; surgical evacuation is usually effective.

Muscle haematomas can occur in any part of the body, however, the most common sites are the iliopsoas muscle and the flexor compartment of the forearm. The muscles in the forearm and the shin are enclosed in tight fascial compartments and even relatively small bleeds can cause a large rise in pressure in the intracompartmental space. Volkmann's contracture of the hand and foot deformities have been reported as a result of such bleeding incidences within the closed compartments. The treatment may be of a conservative nature wherein haemostasis is established, the limb rested in elevation, analgesia provided and as the swelling subsides there will be a decrease in pain and a gradual return of function. Should the pressure be very high, decompression is vital. This decompression may be performed either by drainage of the haematoma or by formal surgery and incision of the fascial envelope. The most common and most serious of the muscle bleeds occurs in the iliopsoas muscle. An iliopsoas haematoma of the right side can mimic appendicitis and care must be taken. Femoral nerve palsy may present as an area of reduced sensation in the anterior aspect of the thigh [12]. Attempts to extend the hip joint causes severe pain and forces the patient into hyperlordosis of the lumbar spine. As it is difficult to clinically differentiate between a bleed into the iliopsoas muscle and an intra-articular haemorrhage into the hip joint, one must rely on further investigations.

CT scans and ultrasonography are the best ways to diagnose and follow up an iliopsoas haematoma to full recovery. The iliopsoas bleed takes a long time to improve and the flexion contracture of the hip joint may persist for weeks. Secondary haemorrhages into the same area are common and hence prophylactic factor replacement is advised. Whereas coxhaemarthoses is a problem of days, an iliopsoas haematoma may require weeks until full recovery is achieved. Up to 18 months of rehabilitation may be necessary for the total recovery of a femoral nerve palsy related to an iliopsoas haematoma.

Pseudotumours are basically encapsulated haematomas. Proximal pseudotumours occur in the proximal skeleton, especially around the femur and pelvis. They appear to originate in the soft tissue, erode bone secondarily from outside, and develop slowly over many years. Proximal pseudotumours occur in adults and do not respond to conservative treatment. They should be removed surgically as soon as they are diagnosed.

Preoperative arterial embolization of such pseudotumours is recommended in order to diminish the size of the lesion and make surgical removal easier.

Distal pseudotumours, occurring distally to the wrist and ankle, appear to be secondary to intraosseous haemorrhage and develop rapidly. They are seen mainly in children and adolescents. They should be treated primarily with long-term replacement therapy and cast immobilization. In children surgical removal or even amputation is indicated when conservative management fails to prevent progression [13]. Percutaneous evacuation should be considered in inoperable advanced pseudotumours. Evacuation is carried out under image intensifier control; the cavity is filled with different quantities of fibrin seal or cancellous bone depending on the size of the pseudotumour. The presence of one or more progressively enlarging masses in the limbs or pelvis of a person with haemophilia should raise the suspicion of a pseudotumour, although chondrosarcoma and liposarcoma have occurred in such patients.

Conclusion

Early treatment of haemophilia is of paramount importance because the immature skeleton is very sensitive to the complications of haemophilia: severe structural deficiencies may develop quickly. Major haemarthroses should be treated aggressively to prevent synovitis and haemophilic arthropathy. In the author's opinion, radioactive synoviorthesis should be the first choice and can be repeated every three months: if after three synoviorthesis treatments the state of the synovitis has not improved sufficiently then arthroscopic or open synovectomy is indicated. At the stage of haemophilic arthropathy possible treatments include joint debridement, osteotomy, arthrodesis and arthroplasty. Horoszowski *et al.* [14] have reported the use of multiple joint procedures on haemophilia patients in a single operative session. This succeeded in achieving a functional limb. The complication rate was less than expected and the rehabilitation period was relatively short. Ragni *et al.* [15] have reported that HIV-infected patients with CD4 counts of 200 mm^3 or less have a 13% rate of postoperative infection. Joint arthroplasty appeared to have 10 times the risk of infection compared to other procedures. For each patient the decision regarding orthopaedic surgery must be individualized and balanced with the potential quality of life benefits afforded by the surgery. When a patient is suffering incapacitating pain, then the improvement of quality of life certainly makes for a situation where the procedure should be performed, provided the patient is fully informed.

References

1 Rodriguez-Merchan EC. Common orthopaedic problems in haemophilia. *Haemophilia* 1999; 5(Suppl 1): 53–60.

2 Rodriguez-Merchan EC. Effects of hemophilia on articulations of children and adults. *Clin Orthop* 1996; 328: 7–13.

3 Rodriguez-Merchan EC, Ribbans WJ. Symposium on prevention and management of chronic hemophilic synovitis. *Clin Orthop* 1997; 343: 6–92.

4 Pettersson H, Gilbert MS. Classification of hemophilic arthropathy. In: Pettersson H, Gilbert MS, eds. *Diagnostic Imaging in Hemophilia*. Berlin: Springer-Verlag, 1985: 56–66.

5 Rodriguez-Merchan EC (editorial). Management of the orthopaedic complications of haemophilia. *J Bone Joint Surg (Br)* 1998; 80–B: 191–6.

6 Löfqvist T, Sanzen L, Petersson C, Nilsson IM. Total hip replacement in patients with hemophilia. 13 hips in 11 patients followed for 1–16 years. *Acta Orthop Scand* 1996; 67: 321–4.

7 Kelley SS, Lachiewicz PF, Gilbert MS, Bolander ME, Jankiewicz JJ. Hip arthroplasty in hemophilic arthropathy. *J Bone Joint Surg (Am)* 1995; 77–A: 828–34.

8 Smith MA, Urquhart DR, Savidge GF. The surgical management of varus deformity in haemophilic arthropathy of the knee. *J Bone Joint Surg (Br)* 1981; 63–B: 261–5.

9 Rodriguez-Merchan EC, Magallon M, Galindo E. Joint debridement for haemophilic arthropathy of the knee. *Int Orthop* 1994; 18: 135–8.

10 Pearce MS, Smith MA, Savidge GF. Supramalleolar osteotomy for haemophilic arthropathy of the ankle. *J Bone Joint Surg (Br)* 1994; 76–B: 947–50.

11 Heim M, Rodriguez-Merchan EC, Horoszowski H. Current trends in hemophilia and other coagulation disorders. Orthopaedic complications and management. *Int J Peditr Hematol/Oncol* 1994; 1: 545–51.

12 Fernandez-Palazzi F, Rivas-Hernandez S, De Bosch N, De Saez AR. Hematomas within the iliopsoas muscles in hemophilic patients. The Latin American experience. *Clin Orthop* 1996; 328: 19–24.

13 Rodriguez-Merchan EC. The haemophilic pseudotumour. *Int Orthop* 1995; 19: 255–60.

14 Horoszowski H, Heim M, Schulman S, Varon D, Martinowitz U. Multiple

joint procedures in a single operative session on hemophilic patients. *Clin Orthop* 1996; 328: 60–4.

15 Ragni MV, Crossett LS, Herndon JH. Postoperative infection following orthopaedic surgery in human immunodeficiency virus-infected hemophiliacs with CD counts <200/mm^3. *J Arthroplasty* 1995; 10: 716–21.

11 Physiotherapy following Orthopaedic Surgery in Haemophilia

Lucy Orr

Introduction

The most common sites of spontaneous bleeding in a person with severe haemophilia are the joints, particularly the knees, elbows and ankles. Intra-articular bleeds result initially in an inflammatory synovitis, but with repeated bleeds chronic destructive changes occur leading eventually to secondary degenerative

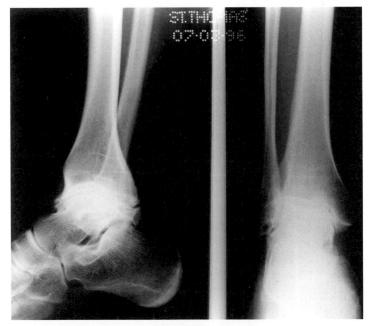

Figure 11.1 Lateral and anteroposterior radiograph showing advanced degenerative changes in the ankle.

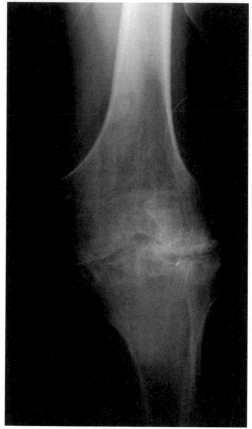

(a)

Figure 11.2
(a) Anteroposterior, and
(b) lateral radiographs showing
advanced degenerative changes
in the knee.

changes at an early age (Figs 11.1 & 11.2). The consequences of
this are significant as several joints are often affected.

Until the mid 1960s orthopaedic surgery was not an option for
people with haemophilia as the risks of bleeding were too great,
but the introduction of factor concentrates made surgery a viable
option and a number of orthopaedic procedures have been, and
continue to be, carried out world-wide. It is not the purpose of
this chapter to describe these procedures in detail, but to provide
an overview of the most common orthopaedic procedures
employed in the care of the patient with haemophilia, so that the
principles of physiotherapy intervention surrounding such procedures can be better understood.

Physiotherapy following elective orthopaedic surgery is largely
dictated by the postoperative protocols of the orthopaedic consultant and will therefore vary between haemophilia centres.

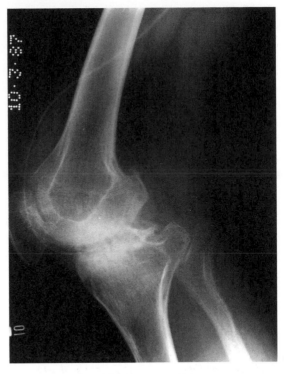

Figure 11.2 *(continued)* (b)

The need for physiotherapy following orthopaedic surgery is however, widely acknowledged and it is possible to provide guidelines for physiotherapy intervention during the orthopaedic episode of care. Issues arising that are pertinent to the individual with haemophilia and their physiotherapist will also be highlighted.

One of the most important considerations is that both orthopaedic surgery and subsequent physiotherapy is essentially the same for a person with haemophilia as for a person without a clotting disorder, provided sufficient levels of the missing factor are maintained throughout the course of treatment [1,2]. Factor replacement should be provided for physiotherapy, if the patient is not on prophylaxis, as well as during the in-patient period.

Indications for orthopaedic surgery

The physiotherapist may well be the person who initially recognizes that an orthopaedic opinion should be sought following the referral of a patient with an increasingly painful joint. The patient may attribute the pain to bleeding into the joint, but closer questioning of the pattern of pain frequently reveals a history of morning stiffness in the joint, a reduced walking distance and increased pain and stiffness after long periods of activity or rest, all of which are indicative of pain that is arthritic in nature rather than the pain of an intra-articular bleed.

Not all bleeding in haemophilia occurs as a result of spontaneous haemorrhage. Patients with an established arthropathy may well complain of bleeding into a joint which is not controlled by factor replacement therapy. This is known as a target joint. At this stage of joint deterioration the apparently spontaneous bleeding may not be caused by too little clotting factor but instead by the secondary arthritis that is a result of previous repeated bleeds. The arthritic changes alter the mechanical stresses on the joint, causing bleeding [3].

Another important consideration is that not all joint problems are haemophilia related and that 'primary orthopaedic conditions can and do occur in patients with haemophilia' [3]. A disc prolapse with referred pain into the ankle can be mistaken for an ankle bleed, or a slipped capital femoral epiphysis could initially be attributed to bleeding into the hip joint. A full history and thorough subjective and physical examination is vital.

If conservative treatment methods such as increased prophylaxis, physiotherapy or splinting are unsuccessful in improving the symptoms of chronic haemophilic arthropathy, then orthopaedic surgery may be the only option remaining. The main indications for orthopaedic surgery are:
• persistent pain or haemorrhage despite adequate factor replacement therapy;
• the presence of a deformity or arthropathy in a joint with symptoms that does not respond to conservative treatment;
• X-ray changes [3,4].

There are several factors unique to the patient with haemophilia that must be considered prior to surgery.
1 *Age of patient.* The process of joint damage may begin at an early age, when the bones are still growing, if bleeding into the joint is not prevented with sufficient factor replacement. The patient who requires orthopaedic surgery is frequently only in their third or fourth decade. All orthopaedic procedures have a limited lifespan and options for revision and further surgery must also be taken into account.

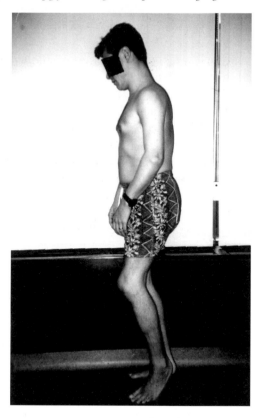

Figure 11.3 The classic pattern of multiple joint involvement in patients with severe haemophilia; fixed flexion deformities of the elbows, hips and knees with ankles plantarflexed.

2 *Multiple joint involvement.* The pattern of bleeding in haemophilia is often into several 'target' joints, with resultant arthropathy in more than one joint. It is possible for an individual with severe haemophilia to present with arthritic changes in a number of joints, as well as deformities produced by extensive muscle bleeds. The classic pattern in the lower limb is one of flexion, with fixed flexion deformities at the hips and knees and plantar flexion at the ankles (Fig. 11.3). Operating on just one joint will not enable the patient to suddenly adopt an upright posture; realistic goals must be set and rehabilitation programmes adapted to take into account any residual deformity.

3 *Loss of joint range.* Loss of range of movement (ROM) can be quite dramatic in a joint affected by chronic haemophilic arthropathy. A patient due to undergo a total knee replacement (TKR), for example, may well have a fixed flexion deformity at the knee of 30° or 40°, far greater than the 'average' patient. Postoperatively, recovery of ROM will therefore be slower and the ideal postoperative range of 0–90° is not always achievable. More important is the reduction or elimination of pain, the cessation of spontaneous bleeding into the joint and an improvement in function.

For surgery to have the greatest chance of success, integrated care by the orthopaedic and haemophilia teams including doctors, nurses and physiotherapists is essential [3–6]. The physiotherapist plays a crucial role in the orthopaedic episode of care [4,7] and without physiotherapy intervention the likelihood of a good functional outcome for the patient is greatly reduced. The motivation and co-operation of the patient is also necessary if the surgical procedure is to be successful.

With any end-stage arthropathy there will be an associated soft tissue contracture. A thorough preoperative assessment will highlight the extent of any contractures, and underlines one of the major differences between haemophilic arthropathy and other joint pathologies.

Preoperative assessment

The following should be noted prior to surgery:
- ROM;
- muscle strength;
- joint circumference;
- mobility and use of walking aids;
- pain;
- extent of any other joint involvement;
- activities of daily living; and
- functional assessment, e.g. Health Assessment Questionnaire.

Prior to surgery, it is important to assess the joints which can refer pain to a region to exclude their involvement. For example, the hip should be assessed prior to knee surgery. A home exercise programme to strengthen muscles or a course of hydrotherapy is often beneficial preoperatively.

The dangers of immobilization are now well recognized, following a bleed, injury or surgery [8,9]. Physiotherapy should start as soon as possible postoperatively. The aims of physiotherapy following orthopaedic surgery are listed below.

Aims of physiotherapy

- Reduce swelling.
- Recover full muscle strength.
- Increase ROM.
- Minimize risk of soft tissue adhesions and shortening.
- Re-educate gait.
- Maximize function.

Orthopaedic procedures and physiotherapy intervention

Synovectomy

A synovectomy may involve the use of radioactive isotopes, or be surgical. A surgical synovectomy may be open or arthroscopic. A synovectomy performed using radioactive isotopes is said to reduce or halt the incidence of spontaneous haemorrhage [4,10], with a shorter period of rehabilitation required than for surgical procedures [4]. Open and arthroscopic synovectomies appear to reduce the number of bleeds but do not slow the progression of the arthropathy [2,4,11–13]; they may also reduce pain [2,13]. Synovectomies should not be performed with the aim of increasing ROM and in fact they may result in a loss of ROM [2–4,10,13,14], particularly in the knee [3,10]. Arthroscopic synovectomies seem to have a less detrimental impact on ROM, with a shorter recovery period [4].

Some authors advocate early active physiotherapy immediately postoperatively [3,13], while others recommend this should start a few days postoperatively [11,12]. Smith [3] suggests the use of the Continuous Passive Movement machine (CPM) in conjunction with active exercises for surgical synovectomy of the knee. Intensive physiotherapy is necessary following synovectomy of the knee because of the tendency to lose ROM postoperatively and this may need to continue for several months with sufficient factor cover.

Tendon lengthening

Tendon lengthening relieves a fixed deformity without loss of muscle function. Hamstring lengthening for fixed flexion deformity of the knee and tendo-achilles lengthening for ankle equinus are the most commonly performed procedures for individuals with haemophilia [3,4,10,14]. An established muscle contracture may be associated with a secondary capsular contracture and so a capsular release may be performed at the same time [3,14]. Although described, they are seldom applicable in patients with haemophilia; soft tissue procedures in the management of fixed deformity are rarely successful.

Postoperatively the limb is immobilized in a splint to maintain the newly acquired length but without adequate active control the contracture will recur [3]. Intensive physiotherapy is therefore vital to help maintain muscle length, improve muscle strength within the newly acquired range, re-educate gait and minimize the formation of scar tissue.

Osteotomy

An osteotomy is a suitable surgical intervention in joints where a deformity can be identified and it can be used to correct that deformity while avoiding intra-articular surgery. This can be a valuable operation due to the often young age of patients with haemophilia presenting for orthopaedic surgery. The extra-articular correction of the deformity allows a more normal load distribution within the joint, thereby relieving mechanical stresses. Despite advanced clinical and radiographic changes a limb that is well aligned appears to function well [4]. The knee and ankle are the most common joints where this procedure is applicable.

Degenerative changes, mainly affecting the medial compartment of the knee joint, are associated with a varus deformity. These are most commonly corrected with a proximal tibial osteotomy [4,10,15]. Changes in the lateral compartment are associated with a valgus deformity and are corrected with a supracondylar femoral osteotomy [4] which can also be used to correct a fixed flexion deformity at the knee [4,10]. The total ROM remains the same but full extension is achieved by 'borrowing' flexion, thereby restoring a more normal functional range [3]. The most common deformities associated with ankle and subtalar joint arthropathy are plantar flexion and valgus deformity at the ankle. This valgus deformity is correctable with a supra-malleolar osteotomy [16].

Results of reported studies demonstrate that osteotomies performed on individuals with haemophilia result in an increase or maintenance of ROM [15], a reduction in the number and severity of spontaneous bleeding episodes [3,15,16], a reduction in pain [16], improved or redeveloped joint space seen on X-ray [15] and a considerable delay in the development of a severe arthropathy [10,15].

Physiotherapy following osteotomy focuses on re-establishing and maintaining the range achieved peroperatively, e.g. gaining full, active extension of a previously fixed flexed knee. From experience, any extension gained passively is soon lost if there is no active control. The CPM is used but it must be for short periods of 2–3 hours only, to allow active exercises to be carried out on a regular basis. Once the stitches have been removed the patient can begin hydrotherapy but this must be accompanied by land sessions under factor cover to ensure ROM is maintained.

The last few degrees of active extension are often difficult to achieve as a longstanding fixed flexion deformity can mean that there will be active insufficiency in the newly available inner range. This, coupled with the fact that the patient is partial weight-bearing (PWB) for six weeks and therefore unable to perform many weight-bearing exercises during that time, results in a long period of rehabilitation.

Patients are generally put into plaster following a proximal or supramalleolar tibial osteotomy for six weeks and are PWB [16]. Physiotherapy, once out of plaster, consists of land sessions and hydrotherapy [15], and must include exercises to improve proprioception.

Total joint replacement

Total hip and knee replacements were some of the first orthopaedic procedures carried out on patients with haemophilia; both reduce pain and the incidence of spontaneous bleeding, but a TKR does not necessarily result in an increase in ROM in patients with haemophilia [2,3,6,7,17]. Total elbow and shoulder replacements are also possible but are performed less frequently. Total ankle replacements are not performed, with ankle arthrodesis being the preferred procedure.

Indications for a total joint replacement are advanced arthropathy as demonstrated by radiographic changes, pain, deformity, restricted ROM or marked functional impairment [4]. The extent of any radiographic change is not always directly related to the symptoms described by the patient. A full clinical assessment taking into account X-rays, pain, number of spontaneous bleeds, ROM and function is necessary prior to surgery.

Adequate pain relief in the postoperative period is essential but may be very difficult to achieve. Large doses of opiates are often required as the patient may be taking opiates for pain relief preoperatively and there is a certain amount of pain with the physiotherapy rehabilitation programme, certainly in the initial stages. Wherever possible, pain relief should be given in anticipation of physiotherapy.

Physiotherapy begins immediately postoperatively and follows a standard protocol, with exercises progressed gradually. Ice is frequently used to reduce swelling. Should a bleed occur, pulsed shortwave can be used to aid the resolution of the bleed. Interferential can also be used if pulsed shortwave is not available.

Following a TKR a standard protocol can be used as a guideline, bearing in mind that the same ROM and level of mobility is not necessarily expected at discharge. This is owing to the extent of the periarticular soft tissue damage associated with the arthropathy and, in many patients, the presence of an arthropathy in other associated joints. Occasionally there may be quadriceps weakness secondary to femoral nerve damage, as a result of a previous iliopsoas haemorrhage. There may also be a residual fixed flexion deformity at the hip. Physiotherapy following a total hip replacement can also follow a standard protocol, always avoiding adduction, internal rotation and flexion beyond 90°, as with any other patient. Hydrotherapy is an excellent form of treatment following joint replacements and other orthopaedic procedures as it enables several joints to be treated at the same time.

Total elbow replacements can be used for haemophilia patients with elbow arthropathy but, because of their fragility and short lifespan, they may not be indicated for patients with lower limb problems where increased use of the upper limbs is required. Two other options have been cited in the literature, the first being a radial head resection with a partial elbow synovectomy. Rodriguez-Merchan *et al.* [11] and Löfquist *et al.* [2] have reported good results with a reduction in spontaneous bleeds [11] and pain [2,11], but no slowing down of the degenerative process [11]. A silastic interposition arthroplasty is the second option. Two studies by Smith *et al.* [18,19] report a reduction in pain and bleeding at a minimum of five years follow-up, plus an increase in ROM. There was a greater improvement in pronation and supination compared with flexion and extension. Physio-therapy is active rather than passive and can include hydrotherapy following the removal of sutures [11,19].

Arthrodesis

Arthrodesis is one of the oldest orthopaedic procedures available, and one of the most successful. It is the surgical intervention of choice for the ankle with end-stage haemophilic arthropathy, pain and bleeding [3,4,7,10,14]. As the arthropathy progresses the ankle may ankylose naturally but the patient often complains of considerable pain with minimal movement. Surgical fusion of the joint therefore leaves the patient no worse off than preoperatively in terms of ROM but with the benefits of being pain free. Arthrodesis is not indicated where there is a significant ROM. A below-knee plaster is *in situ* for three months postoperatively and the patient is non-weight-bearing for the first two months. Physiotherapy involves gait re-education and exercises for the muscles around the hip and knee while in plaster. Once out of plaster physiotherapy to improve muscle strength and proprioception around the ankle can begin.

An arthrodesis can also be used for the shoulder, wrist, sub-talar joint and occasionally the hip and knee [4,7]. Arthrodesis of the knee may produce secondary changes in the contralateral knee and is not indicated if the contralateral knee is already affected by arthropathy. However, it may be the only option following failure of a prosthesis.

Fracture management

Fractures occur in the haemophilia population as in any other patient and their incidence may be increasing as advances in haematological care enable people with haemophilia to lead more active lives. The management will be similar to the non-haemophilic population but should be carried out in conjunction with the haemophilia unit so that initial haemostasis can be achieved quickly and maintained [3,4]. There is no greater incidence of excessive bleeding, non-union or other complications such as compartment syndromes in patients with haemophilia following fractures. If the fracture occurs close to a joint with pre-existing haemophilic arthropathy then care must be taken to ensure that fracture management does not further compromise the joint [3].

Fracture management was at one time largely conservative in patients with haemophilia, but with the ability to control bleeding, improved surgical techniques and a greater awareness of the benefits of active mobilization, normal orthopaedic principles can be applied. Internal and external fixation are the first choice of treatment, enabling rehabilitation of the soft tissues to begin without delay.

Compartment syndrome

Compartment syndromes occurring in haemophilia are unusual and when they do occur are the result of local intramuscular bleeding. The most common sites are the iliopsoas, calf and forearm. The primary course of treatment is immediate factor replacement therapy, followed quickly by physiotherapy to reduce the swelling and relieve pressure on the nerve where this is possible, once haemostasis has been achieved [3].

Conclusion

Physiotherapy is an important part of the orthopaedic episode of care for patients with haemophilia. Patient motivation and close co-operation between the members of the multidisciplinary team is also needed in order to provide the patient with the best opportunity for a good outcome. If adequate factor levels are maintained then physiotherapy intervention is largely the same for individuals with haemophilia as for those without a clotting disorder. Certain issues do need to be considered, however, such as the age of the patient, the extent of the joint damage with associated soft tissue contracture and the likelihood of multiple joint involvement. With these issues in mind a thorough pre-operative assessment including subjective, physical and functional measurements is required, and realistic goals must be set with the patient. This will facilitate the best outcome for any surgical procedure.

References

1 Cotta S, Jutras M, McQuarrie A. *Physical Therapy in Haemophilia*. The National Hemophilia Foundation and the Canadian Haemophilia Society, New York, 1986.

2 Löfqvist T, Nilsson IM, Petersson C. Orthopaedic surgery in hemophilia. 20 years' experience in Sweden. *Clin Orthop* 1996; 332: 232–41.

3 Smith MA. Orthopedic management of hemophilia. In: Savidge GF, Seghatchian G, eds. *Factor VIII — Von Willebrand Factor*, Vol. II. Boca Raton: CRC Press, 1989: 183–220.

4 Gilbert MS, Wiedel JD. *The Treatment of Hemophilia — Current Orthopedic Management*. New York: The National Hemophilia Foundation, 1996.

5 DeGnore LT, Wilson FC. Surgical management of hemophilic arthropathy. *Instr Course Lect* 1989; 38: 383–8.

6 Karthaus RP, Novakova IRO. Total knee replacement in haemophilic arthropathy. *J Bone Joint Surg* 1988; 70–B: 382–5.

7 Smith MA. Orthopaedics: current practice. *The Bulletin*. London: The Haemophilia Society, 1990; 13–15.

8 Evans P. The healing process at cellular level: a review. *Physiotherapy* 1980; 66: 256–9.

9 Videman T. Connective tissue and immobilisation: key factors in musculoskeletal degeneration? *Clin Orthop* 1987; 221: 26–32.

10 Rodriguez-Merchan EC. Management of the orthopaedic complications of haemophilia. *J Bone Joint Surg* 80–B: 191–6, 1998.

11 Rodriguez-Merchan EC, Galindo E, Magallon M, Gago J, Villar A, Sanjurjo MJ. Resection of the radial head and partial open synovectomy of the elbow in the young adult with haemophilia: long-term results. *Haemophilia* 1995; 1: 262–6.

12 Rodriguez-Merchan EC, Galindo E, Ladreda JMM, Pardo JA. Surgical synovectomy in haemophilic arthropathy of the knee. *Int Orthop* 1994; 18: 38–41.

13 Teigland JC, Tjonnfjord GE, Evensen SA, Charania B. Synovectomy for haemophilic arthropathy: 6–21 years of follow-up in 16 patients. *J Intern Med* 1994; 235: 239–43.

14 Ribbans WJ, Phillips M, Stock D, Stibe E. Haemophilic ankle problems: orthopaedic solutions. *Haemophilia* 1995; 1: 91–6.

15 Smith MA, Urquhart DR, Savidge GF. The surgical management of varus deformity in haemophilic arthropathy of the knee. *J Bone Joint Surg* 1981; 63–B: 261–5.

16 Pearce MS, Smith MA, Savidge GF. Supramalleolar tibial osteotomy for haemophilic arthropathy of the ankle. *J Bone Joint Surg* 1994; 76–B: 947–50.

17 Thomason HC, Wilson FC, Lachiewicz PF, Kelley SS. Knee arthroplasty in hemophilic arthropathy. *Clin Orthop* 1999; 360: 169–73.

18 Butler-Manuel PA, Smith MA, Savidge GF. Silastic interposition for haemophilic arthropathy of the elbow. *J Bone Joint Surg* 1990; 72–B: 472–4.

19 Smith MA, Savidge GF, Fountain EJ. Interposition arthroplasty in the management of advanced haemophilic arthropathy of the elbow. *J Bone Joint Surg* 1983; 65–B: 436–40.

12 Rehabilitation in Developing Countries

Lily Heijnen and Muhammad Tariq Sohail

Introduction

There is no substantial literature on the subject of rehabilitation of haemophilia patients in developing countries. A literature search in Medline from 1966 to January 1999 yielded two articles: one on prophylactic therapy programmes in developing countries [1] and a bulletin of the World Health Organization, describing modern treatment of haemophilia [2].

Haemophilia care, and especially rehabilitation after muscle and joint bleeds, requires thoroughly trained personnel, well equipped centres and a ready source of virus free factor VIII and IX and other therapeutic material. Educated, co-operative and motivated patients, their relatives and support personnel are imperative for the successful outcome of the problem. In developing countries low literacy rate, lack of awareness, very limited funds, poverty and very few trained technicians and haemophilia comprehensive care centres make treatment and rehabilitation of patients with haemophilia a very difficult and daunting task. The psychosocial taboos, beliefs and inter-family marriages have their own part to play in magnifying the problem of haemophilia care [3].

The World Federation of Haemophilia (WFH) has focused on this subject in the World Congresses. Carol Kasper [4] stated in 1994 that establishment or improvement of haemophilia treatment in a developing country requires goodwill, hard work, creative thinking, co-operation and patience.

A society of concerned patients, parents and physicians can provide the needed energy. Education is the first step in treatment, which should include specific exercise programmes especially for youths. The funding of haemophilia care is a major challenge, but some creative schemes have borne fruit. Experts from the developing countries [5–10] hold similar views.

The magnitude of the problem

It is estimated that 80% of persons with haemophilia world-wide do not have access to adequate medical care [11] and only 20% have access to facilities which are in accordance with the 'state of the art'. In this chapter India and Pakistan will be cited as examples of developing countries.

India has a population of over 900 million so, theoretically, there should be at least 90 000 haemophilia patients in this country. However, there are only four comprehensive care centres (Vellore, Delhi, Mumbai and Pune) and the Haemophilia Federation of India (HFI) has about 5000 registered persons with haemophilia, who get their treatment via the 50 chapters which are organized in different cities all over the country. The HFI raises money and imports most of the factor concentrates that are used in the country. (Kaul V., personal communication 1999). In Pakistan the situation is similar and for a population of 130 million the estimated number of patients with haemophilia is around 13 000. Some patients are registered at university and private hospitals [12]. Although the number of patients getting help and guidance through haemophilia patients' welfare societies is still very low, these societies have to put an enormous effort into raising funds to provide safe therapeutic clotting material. Lately, awareness of the importance of patient education, exercises and physiotherapy is also gaining momentum [13].

Treatment options

In developing countries, society in general, health authorities and health professionals are confronted with major problems which make it difficult to raise interest and awareness of such a rare disorder as haemophilia. The population in most developing countries is heterogeneous, having a three tier society in relation to income, education and motivation. 80% is illiterate and has no or a minimal income, 15% has some education and a job and 5% has advanced education and are rich. The best haemophilia care appropriate and possible for each level of the population has to be carefully planned [8].

The development of comprehensive haemophilia care centres including facilities for treatment of musculoskeletal problems will be a long-term goal. Regional reference centres should work in association with the National Haemophilia Societies. The World Federation of Haemophilia has initiated several programmes to assist those in developing countries: training of those involved in haemophilia care like orthopaedic surgeons, physiatrists and physiotherapists; organizing local workshops and the Haemophilia Care Centre twinning programme [11]. Much energy is invested in organizing laboratory diagnosis and safe factor replacement therapy [14]. However, many people with haemophilia from vast countries like India and Pakistan live too far away to benefit from the existence of the centres and/ or cannot afford to pay for replacement therapy.

Prevention of joint and muscle bleeding and its sequels has been accomplished in various countries by prophylactic administration of clotting factors in childhood. But this is very expensive and difficult in developing countries. Home treatment is only available to a few. Rehabilitation on the other hand is inexpensive and efficient; muscle strengthening exercises performed with care need not provoke bleeding.

Treatment protocols have been developed for the management of acute joint and muscle bleeds in situations with a shortage of clotting materials [14].

Education of people with haemophilia and their families, to make them as self-supporting as possible on one hand and using existing health services and especially rehabilitation facilities on the other hand, is very important. Of the generally disabled population in India 78% lives in rural areas [15]. The possibilities for community-based rehabilitation are described by Helander *et al.* [16]. This includes a guide for local supervisors, a guide for people with disabilities as well as for schoolteachers and training packages.

For the manufacturing of splints, crutches and shoe adaptations, local materials are preferred over 'high tech' imported materials as the first serve their purpose as well as the last.

Different aspects of rehabilitation in haemophilia which are, of course, also applicable in developing countries are described in books [17,18] and recent articles by Buzzard [19] and Heijnen and De Kleijn [20]. In this chapter an overview of treatment is outlined.

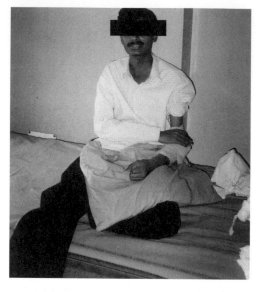

Figure 12.1 Adolescent with acute elbow bleed being treated with ice.

Acute haemarthrosis

1 Give clotting factor intravenously, if available.

2 Rest the affected arm or leg in a comfortable position with the help of a cushion, padded splint or sling.

3 Give local ice application 15–20 min every 2 hours (Fig. 12.1).

4 Give oral analgesics (no aspirin) and muscle relaxing medication like valium.

5 Provide compression of the joint with a bandage.

6 Limit activities and weight bearing of the lower limb using crutches.

As soon as the bleeding has stopped and pain subsides (without factor replacement this happens in 5–7 days) active movement of the involved limb and muscle strengthening exercises, preferably under supervision of a physiotherapist, should begin. At first exercises should be isometric followed by isotonic, active assisted and isokinetic exercises. As muscle strength improves, in most cases range of motion improves accordingly. If this is not the case active mobilizing exercises are indicated, especially muscle stretching exercises of the antagonists of the atrophic muscles. These stretching exercises should always be done actively by the patient. If full recovery of range of motion is not attained, manual traction or traction with weights can be instituted. When range of motion and muscle strength have improved, training of stability and coordination should be started followed by functional (ADL) exercises. Splints and orthoses are useful if joint instability and/or lack of coordination has been identified.

Special problems

1 Elbow joint. Loss of supination and pronation in combination with loss of extension.

Advise: concentrate on muscle strengthening of the triceps in combination with stretching exercises of the biceps using a pronation-flexion/supination-extension pattern.

2 Knee joint. Impaired motion of the patella causes loss of function.

Advise: Active movement of the patella should commence as soon as possible. If restricted patellar motion persists, cranial and caudal mobilizations should be performed passively. This should not be painful. When dorsal subluxation of the proximal tibia is present, there will be lengthening of the patellar ligament and shortening of the hamstrings. These complications should be taken into account when trying to restore extension. Furthermore, specific attention should be given to rehabilitation of the vastus medialis oblique which is important in control and tracking of the patella.

3 Ankle joint. Loss of dorsiflexion is often compensated by a valgus position and pronation of the foot or by compensatory hyperextension of the knee.

Advise: If dorsiflexion cannot be regained by means of exercises, a heel raise of the shoe should be considered.

When assessing patients with recurrent haemarthroses in one joint, a full assessment of the musculoskeletal system should be made because elbow bleeds may be caused by weakness of the lower limb muscles or a painful knee with limited range of motion, in which case the arms are frequently used to rise from a chair.

Chronic synovitis

In the first place chronic synovitis is managed with active muscle strengthening exercises and splinting in case of instability. Physiotherapy treatment consists of manual traction; rhythmic manually resisted exercises for the main antagonist muscles; joint stability training in non-weight bearing positions.

During a period of major swelling, joint instability and quadriceps weakness crutches should be used during walking, or an anterior opened-thigh splint [21].

The exercises should also be done several times daily at home for 6 weeks to 3 months; combined with icing of the inflamed joint 3–6 times daily; (i.e. ice cube massage for 5–10 min).

If this treatment fails and intensive prophylactic factor replacement therapy is not available, effective alternative ablation of the synovium has to be considered. This objective can be accomplished by chemical or radiotherapeutic measures. Chemical synovectomy was originally described using osmic acid. Rifampicin has been used intra-articularly with very good results [22]. Both osmic acid and Rifampicin produce subsynovial fibrosis and sclerosis of the venous plexus, thus reducing the size of the hypertrophied synovium and reducing the number of bleeding episodes. Rifampicin synovectomy is advantageous being safe and not aggressive to the patient, can be repeated if necessary and does not prevent the use of surgery or radiotherapy. It is also very economical and can be performed on an out-patient basis. It has been shown that patients who underwent this procedure have less radiological changes than the patients who persisted with chronic synovitis.

Synoviorthesis with Yttrium-90 is also effective, but has disadvantages concerning availability, half-life time and the need of specialists familiar with handling these materials.

Arthroscopic (or open) synovectomy can be carried out in certain situations, but this requires a comprehensive haemophilia care team and a large amount of antihaemophilic factors both during and after the surgery and during rehabilitation (which may be difficult and prolonged in the case of an open synovectomy) [23].

Muscle haemorrhage

1 Clotting factor if available.
2 Rest and immobilization with cushions, a padded splint or sling.
3 Analgesics (no aspirin).
4 Ice application 15–20 min every 2 hours.
5 Limit activities and weight bearing of the lower limb using crutches or a wheelchair.

When the bleeding has stopped careful active movement preferably beginning in the hydrotherapy pool, followed by an extensive exercise programme (starting with isometric followed by isotonic, active assisted and isokinetic programmes). Muscle stretching exercises are important to regain muscle fibre length and should be done actively, but slowly by the patient, and should not cause any pain. Furthermore gentle friction can be helpful to prevent contractures caused by scar issue. Deep friction may also be given by an experienced physiotherapist with care and caution and preferably under cover of replacement therapy to prevent rebleeding.

A complication of a muscle haemorrhage can be a compression of a nerve. An iliopsoas bleed may be associated with compression of the femoral nerve which may cause quadriceps weakness. A brace may be necessary to stabilize the knee.

Chronic arthropathy

A full assessment of the patient should be performed because hardly ever is only one joint troubling the patient, although this may be the initial impression. Impairment of one joint influences not only the affected limb but also the contralateral side. Moreover, contractures in ankles, knees and hips may cause increased lordosis and back pain. Impairments of the legs may also aggravate upper limb problems. To enable the patient to start exercising pain reduction is a must. Manual traction, cold or heat application and ultrasound or transcutaneous electrice nerve stimulation (TENS) [24,25] can be applied. Traction can be taught to the patient and his family members either by applying traction distal to the joint involved, for instance with a weight, or by teaching the family member how to perform manual traction. In haemophilic arthropathy the primary aim of traction should be pain reduction and not improvement of range of motion. Once pain reduction is achieved active muscle strengthening and stretching exercises can be started, followed by joint stability training, postural and gait training and functional training. Due to loss of function there is almost invariably a weakness of extensor muscles and shortening of flexor muscles. When the patient does exercises at home it is important to explain which muscle groups should be strengthened and which ones stretched.

Corrective devices in treatment of articular contractures

In case of a flexion contracture of the knee an extension de-subluxation hinge device can be used which is said to prevent the problem of posterior subluxation of the tibia during correction [21].

Serial casting may also be applied. Complications include skin necrosis, cartilage compression and joint subluxation [26]. The disadvantage of serial casting moreover, is that during the casting period active muscle strengthening exercises are hardly feasible and when the plaster is taken off the muscle strength around the joint may not be sufficient to prevent new bleeding episodes. Once the casting has been removed a backsplint or brace should be used until muscle strength is regained and the patient can be mobilized without the danger of an acute bleeding episode due to instability of the joint.

Disabilities

Once the sequelae of recurrent bleeding in muscle and joints have led to disabilities, one should aim at giving the patient functional independence for ambulation and daily activities. Individual patients may need braces, shoe adaptations, special shoes or other orthoses to assist during walking, ADL and work. Special crutches and ambulatory devices are helpful (Fig. 12.2).

Chronic pain associated with these disabilities is often a common complaint. Abuse of analgesics is not uncommon. Secondary degenerative changes in the joints along with the muscle atrophy, shortening of a limb and contractures may all contribute to persistent pain and disability. This produces marked psychological problems, so use of antidepressants and psychological counselling can be helpful.

Education

Even people with haemophilia in developing countries who are diagnosed and are able to visit a doctor when they have a joint or muscle bleed or haemophilia related musculoskeletal problems may not be referred to a rehabilitation service or physiotherapist. This may occur not only because the facility is not available but also, because in some developing countries, even more than in

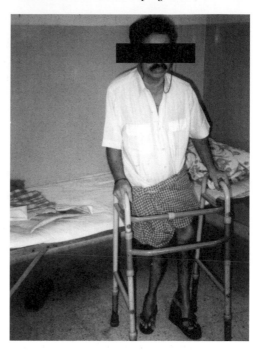

Figure 12.2 Patient with severe joint problems using walking frame and shoe raise.

the western world, the haematologists seem to be focused on replacement therapy and if this is not available they may advise rest and ice but no physical therapy. Therefore education of healthcare workers, people with haemophilia and their families is of the utmost importance. Due to the scarcity of replacement therapy, financial aspects and travel distances, patients will tend to stay at home with 'ordinary' bleeding prob-lems. There is an important role for National Haemophilia Societies and the local chapters, alongside the education that the established comprehensive care centres are able to provide to healthcare workers. Parents and patients should not only be convinced that active muscle strengthening exercises after each bleeding episode are important, but also that trying to obtain the best overall physical condition is very important. Preventing and treating impairments in an early stage is the only way to prevent disabilities and handicaps. Simple leaflets describing treatment strategies and exercises should be produced in the local language with pictures that look familiar to those who will be reading them. The Haemophilia Federation of India and the Haemophilia Patients Welfare Society of Pakistan have developed booklets in, respectively,

Hindi and Urdu and the World Federation and patients' organizations in Europe and the USA and also many haemophilia centres can also provide examples of education material which can be translated and adapted to the local situation. In 1998 for example, a booklet with exercises written by the author in English was translated into Urdu (the official language of Pakistan) [27].

Conclusion

For effective rehabilitation of patients with haemophilia in developing countries it is of utmost importance to educate the patients and their close relatives in early recognition and care of bleeding episodes, and teach simple and effective measures to control bleeding and to restore muscle and joint function. The importance of exercises cannot be over emphasized, as has been said 'Use it or lose it!'.

References

1 Willoughby ML. Prophylactic therapy programs for hemophilia in developing countries. *Pediatr Hematol Oncol* 1997; 14(2): ix–xii.

2 Berntorp E, Boulyjenkov V, Brettler D *et al.* Modern Treatment of haemophilia. *Bull World Health Organ* 1995; 73(5): 691–701.

3 Sohail MT. Hemophilic arthropathy. *JPOA* 1999; 11(1): 50–4.

4 Kasper CK. Treatment of hemophilia in developing countries. *XXI International Congress WFH, Mexico City; April 24–29, 1994.* Book of abstracts, p. 2.

5 Kim KY. Development and maintenance of hemophilia care programme in Korea. *SE Asian J Trop Med Pub Health* 1993; 24(suppl. 1): 52–60.

6 Chuansumrit A. Hemophilia care in Thailand. *XXI International Congress WFH, Mexico City; April 24–29, 1994.* Book of abstracts, p. 23.

7 Camacho B. Haemophilia care in Colombia. *XXI. International Congress WFH, Mexico City; April 24–29, 1994.* Book of abstracts, p. 22.

8 Chandy M. Haemophilia care in developing countries. *XXII International Congress WFH Dublin, Ireland 1996, 23–28 June. Haemophilia* 1996; 2(Suppl. 1): 1.

9 Kavakli K, Nisli G, Polat A *et al.* Clinical severity, therapy models and joint evaluation for hemophilia in a developing country. *XXIII International Congress WFH Haemophilia* 1998; 4(3): 220.

10 Diop S, Thiam D, Badiane M *et al.* Articular complications of hemophilia in Senegal. *Haemophilia Vol* 1998; 4 (3): 218.

11 Lee CA. Towards achieving global haemophilia care-WFH programmes. *Haemophilia* 1998; 4(4): 463–73.

12 Shamsi TS, Oureshi Kh, Ahmed S *et al.* Haemophilic arthropathy in Pakistani patients. *Haemophilia* 1998; 4(3): 219.

13 Sohail MT. Proceeding of 12th International Conference of POA, Bhurban, Pakistan, 1997.

14 Srivastava A, Chuansumrit A, Chandy M, Duraiswamy G, Karagus C. Management of haemophilia in the developing world. *Haemophilia* 1998; 4(4): 474–80.

15 Poonekar PD, Prabhat KG. A look at health care and prosthetic/orthotic services in India. *ONP Business World* 1999; Winter: 24–30.

16 Helander E, Mendis P, Nelson G, Goerdt A. *Training in the Community for People with Disabilities.* Geneva: World Health Organization, 1989.

17 Rizzo Batististella L, Heijnen L. *Rehabilitation in haemophilia.* May 1998. Medifax Int. Brighton, UK.

18 Heijnen L. *Recent Advantages in Rehabilitation in Haemophilia.* Medicine Education Network. Hove, England, 1995.

19 Buzzard BM. Physiotherapy for the prevention of articular contraction in haemophilia. *Haemophilia* 1999; 5(suppl. 1): 10–15.

20 Heijnen L, De Kleijn P. Physiotherapy for the treatment of articular contractures in haemophilia. *Haemophilia* 1999; 5(Suppl. 1): 16–19.

21 Boone DC. Common musculoskeletal problems and their management. In: Boone DC, ed. *Comprehensive Management of Hemophilia.* Philadelphia: FA Davis Company, 1976: 53–85.

22 Caviglia HA, Fernandez-Palazzi F, Maffei E *et al.* Chemical synoviorthesis for hemophilia synovitis. *Clin Orth Rel Res* 1997; 343: 30–6.

23 Sohail MT. Hemophilic arthropathy-experience with intra articular Rifampicin injection. Proceedings of 12th WPOA Meeting, Japan, 1998.

24 Rizzo Battistella L. Rehabilitation in haemophilia — options in the developing world. *Haemophilia* 1998; 4: 486–90.

25 Martinowitz U, Heim M, Navon S. The use of transcutaneous electrice nerve stimulation (TENS) in the treatment of the haemophiliaís. *Rehabilitation Haemophilia* 1989; 5: 15–20.

26 Rodriguez-Merchan EC. Therapeutic options in the management of articular contractures in haemophiliacs. *Haemophilia* 1999; 5(suppl. 1): 5–9.

27 Heijnen L. *Use It Or Lose It.* Haemophilia Patients Welfare Society, Karachi, Pakistan; 1998.

Index